CW00337565

Fast
exercise

igloobooks

igloobooks

Published in 2014
by Igloo Books Ltd
Cottage Farm
Sywell
NN6 0BJ
www.igloobooks.com

The measurements used are approximate.

FIR003 1014
2 4 6 8 10 9 7 5 3 1
ISBN 978-1-78440-139-9

Printed and manufactured in China

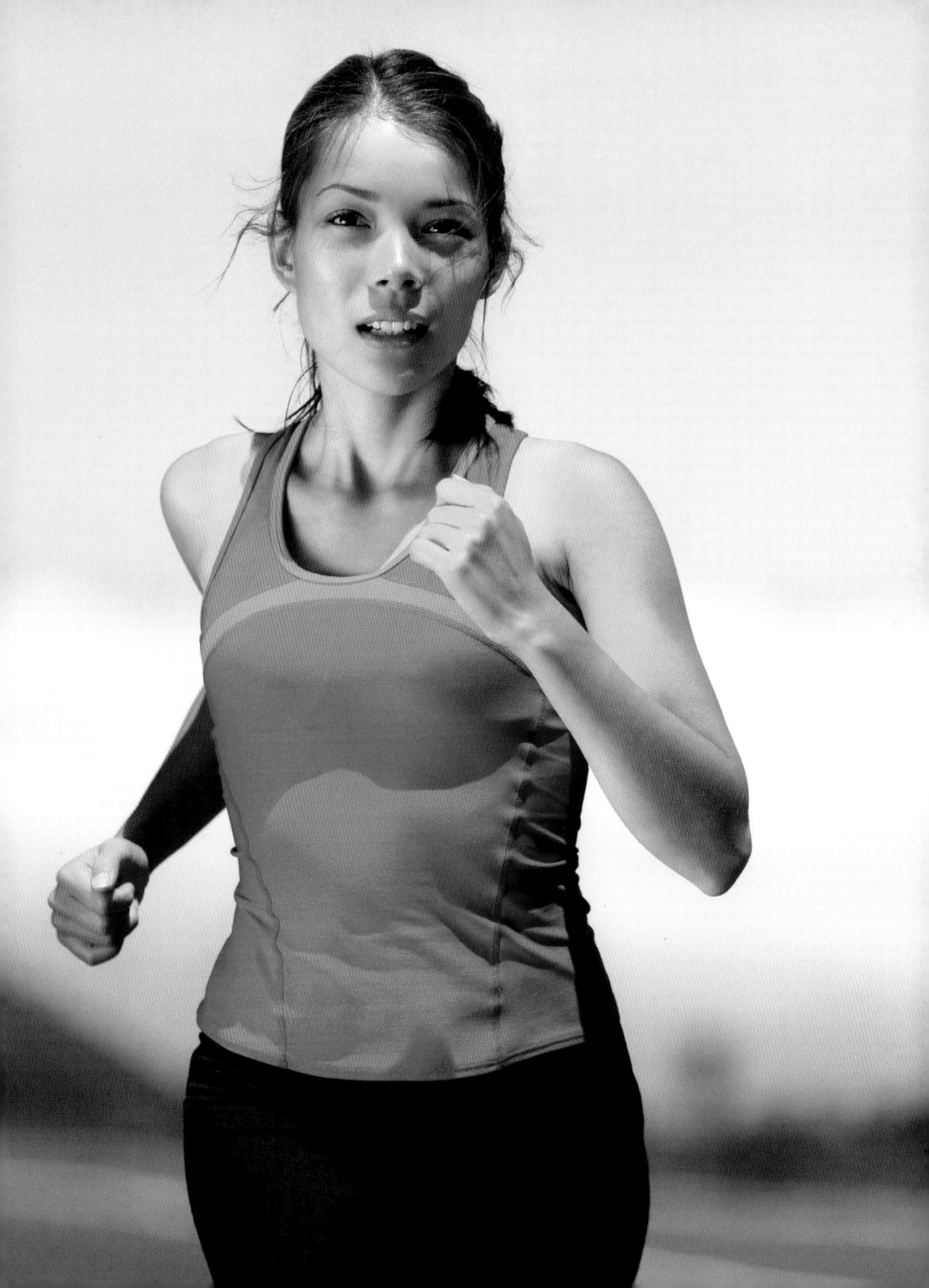

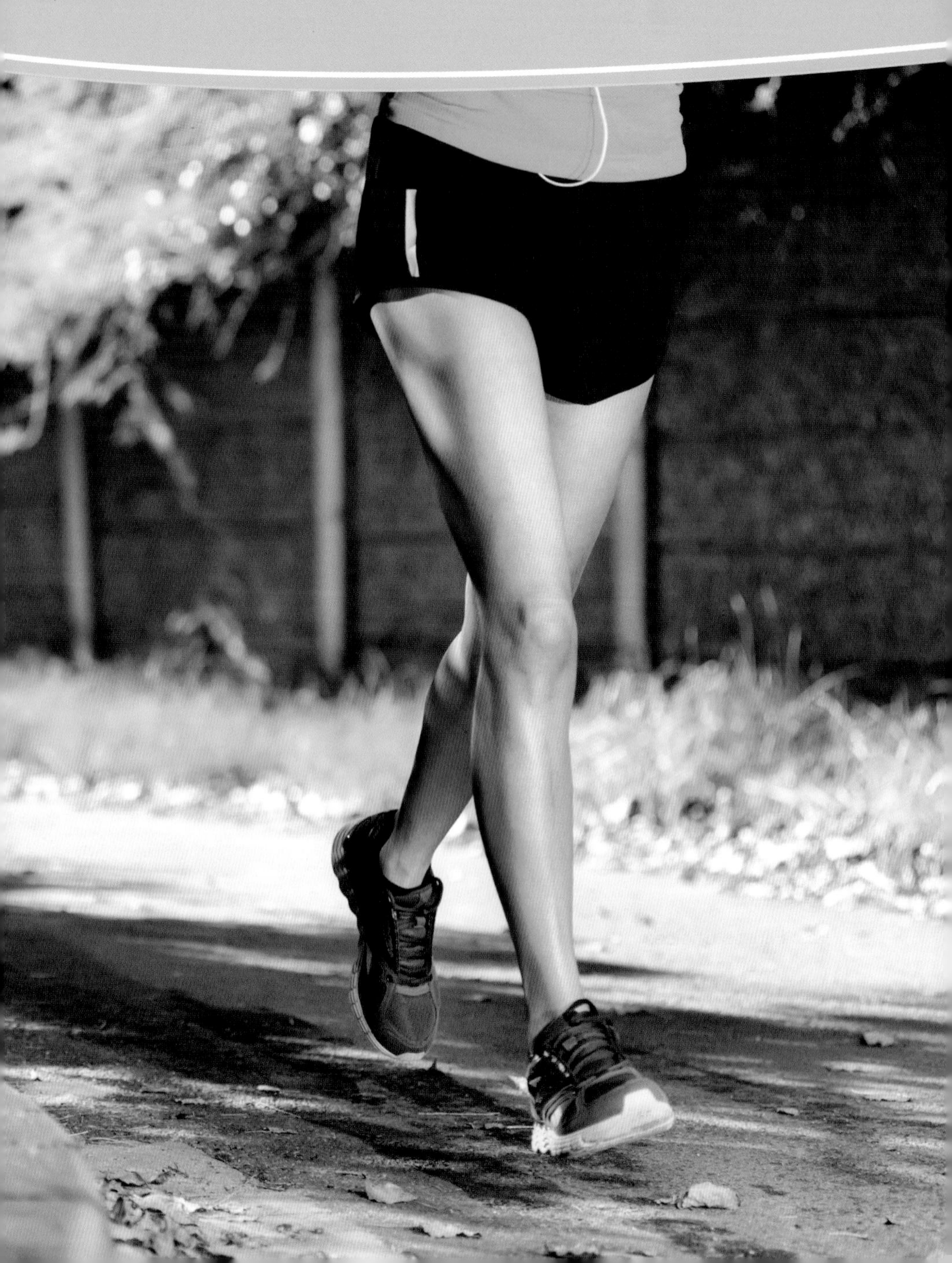

Contents

Introduction

Fast Fitness 6
Why Fit Fast? 8
Fast Fit Works 10
Science of Fast Fitness 14
Health Aware 16
How to Use This Book 18
Fast Fit Ready 22
Get Drinking 26

Exercises

Fast Fitness Choices 28
Running 30
Cycling 38
Swimming 46
Circuits 54
Weighty Work 62
Walking 68
Quick Fix 72
Kickbox 82
Moving Fast 86
Mix It Up 88

Keep It Going

Make It Work 90
Fast Fit Food 94
Calorie Check 98
Exercise Plans 100
Diary Tracker 112
Major Muscles 120
Keep It Fast 122

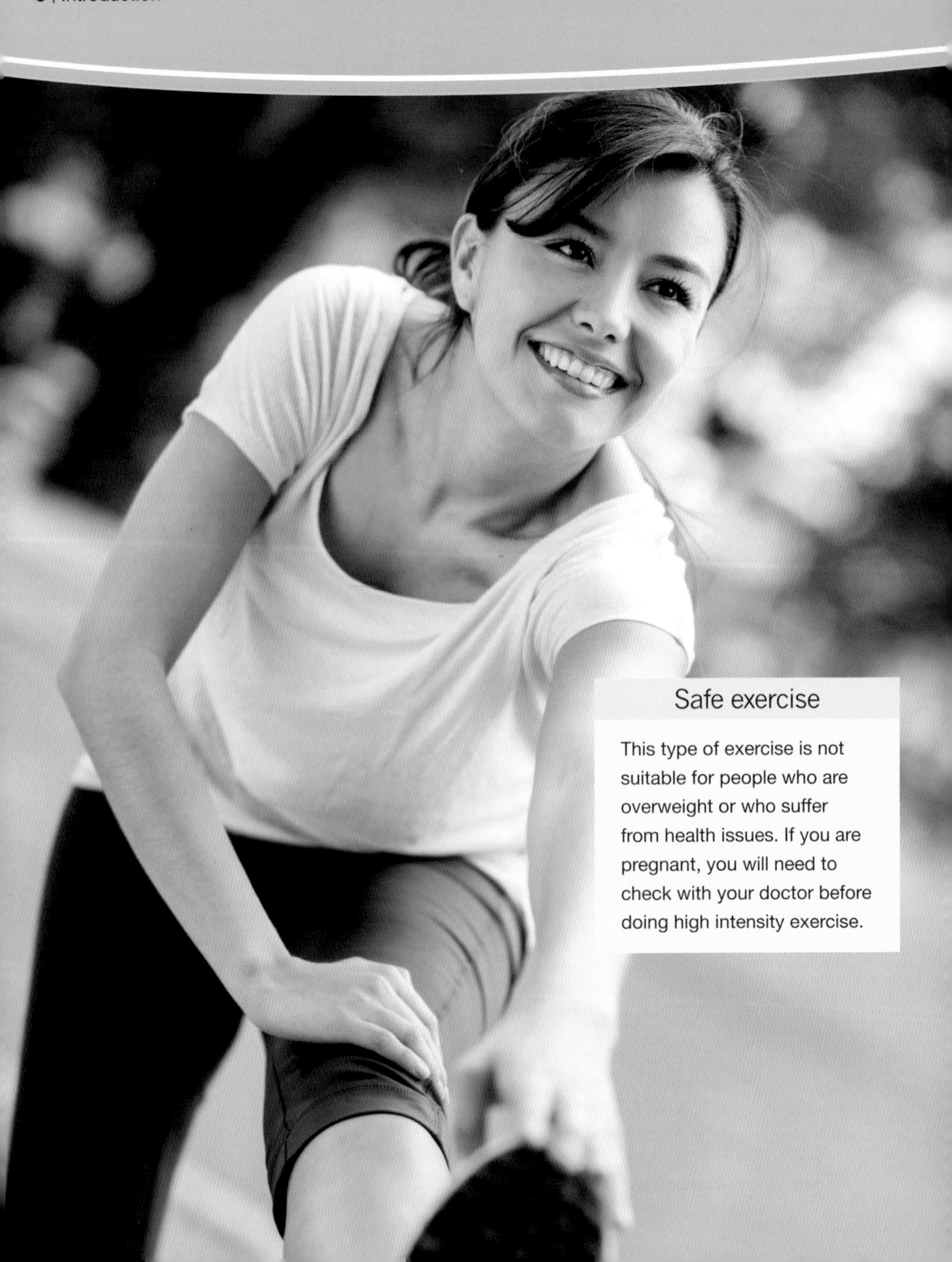

Safe exercise

This type of exercise is not suitable for people who are overweight or who suffer from health issues. If you are pregnant, you will need to check with your doctor before doing high intensity exercise.

Fast Fitness

Do you want to get fit but don't have much time and don't want to spend hours on a treadmill or in the gym? This is the book for you.

We all want to look good and enjoy our bodies, but how can we do that when we don't have the time to spend four hours on fitness a week? Fast fitness is the answer. Read on to find out how you can spend literally minutes on a serious and challenging exercise programme. But be warned – it is not for the faint-hearted!

Fast fitness is training at high intensity. It is about getting fit with short, power-packed bursts of exercise. And by short, we mean short – as in minutes. This is the new effective way to lose weight and get fit.

You can adapt fast fitness to different activities and sports, and to different environments. You do not need special equipment or an expensive gym membership. All you need is determination, commitment and a few minutes a week. It's easy to incorporate into your week and, because it's so wonderfully short, you won't lose motivation to continue.

This book gives you all the information you need to introduce high intensity exercise into your life. As well as workouts that will push your fitness levels to the max, there are targeted exercises for bums, tums and other troublesome areas, and routines that everyone can adapt to their needs.

There's also advice on the best healthy eating plan to support your fitness regime, and tips on ways to make fast fitness a long-term plan rather than a one-day wonder.

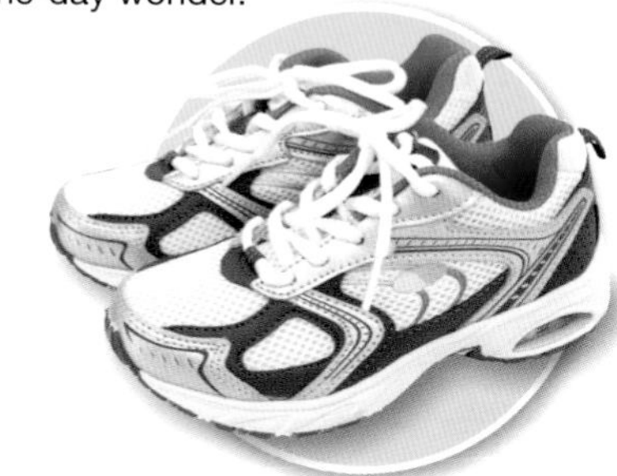

Why Fit Fast?

Who has the time to spend hours running or swim endlessly up and down a pool? Not many women today, that's for sure. We are too busy juggling careers, family and friends. Let's be honest, committing to regular 40-minute sessions of exercise in a class or gym starts off with the best intentions but then there is a deadline at work, you have to cover someone else who is on leave or one of the children is poorly at home...

It is so dispiriting looking at magazines illustrated with photographs of women with fantastically toned bodies demonstrating exercise regimes that seem to require a rigid military campaign for success – each of which takes over 40 minutes a day. How can we get fit when we don't have 40 minutes a day to spare?

Don't despair, because fast fitness could be the answer you're looking for. These short bursts of exercise make you feel good (once you have done them!) and have been shown to be more beneficial than longer workouts in helping you to lose weight and build toned muscles.

The short fitness plans and exercises in this book allow you to fit effective workouts into your busy day. The workouts are a combination of aerobic and anaerobic – designed to help you tone your body, develop a stronger heart and look good. It will feel hot and sweaty but it will be worth it! You don't need to go to a gym or try to keep pace with a DVD. You can work out pretty much wherever you are, and whenever you want.

And the best news of all – it works.

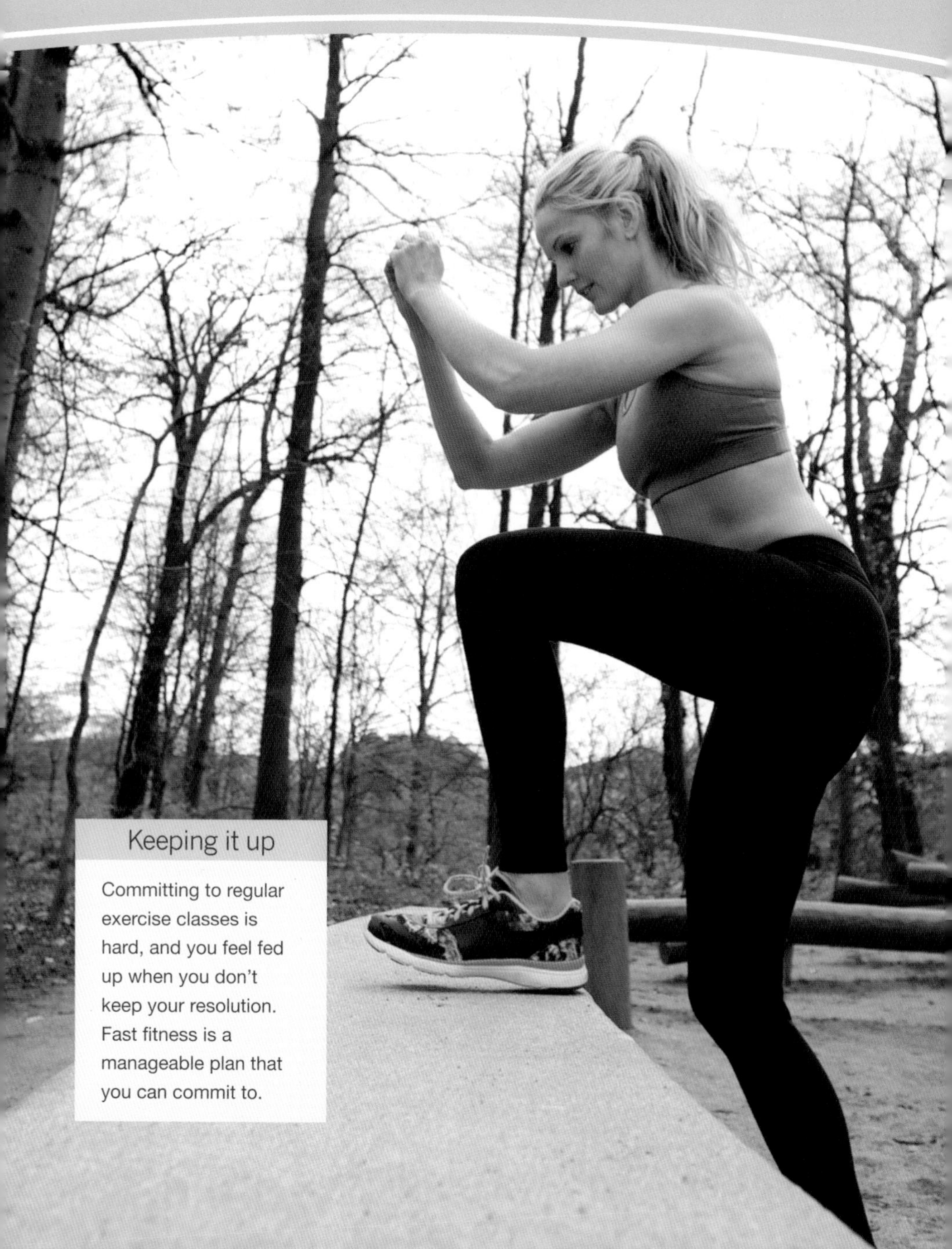

Keeping it up

Committing to regular exercise classes is hard, and you feel fed up when you don't keep your resolution. Fast fitness is a manageable plan that you can commit to.

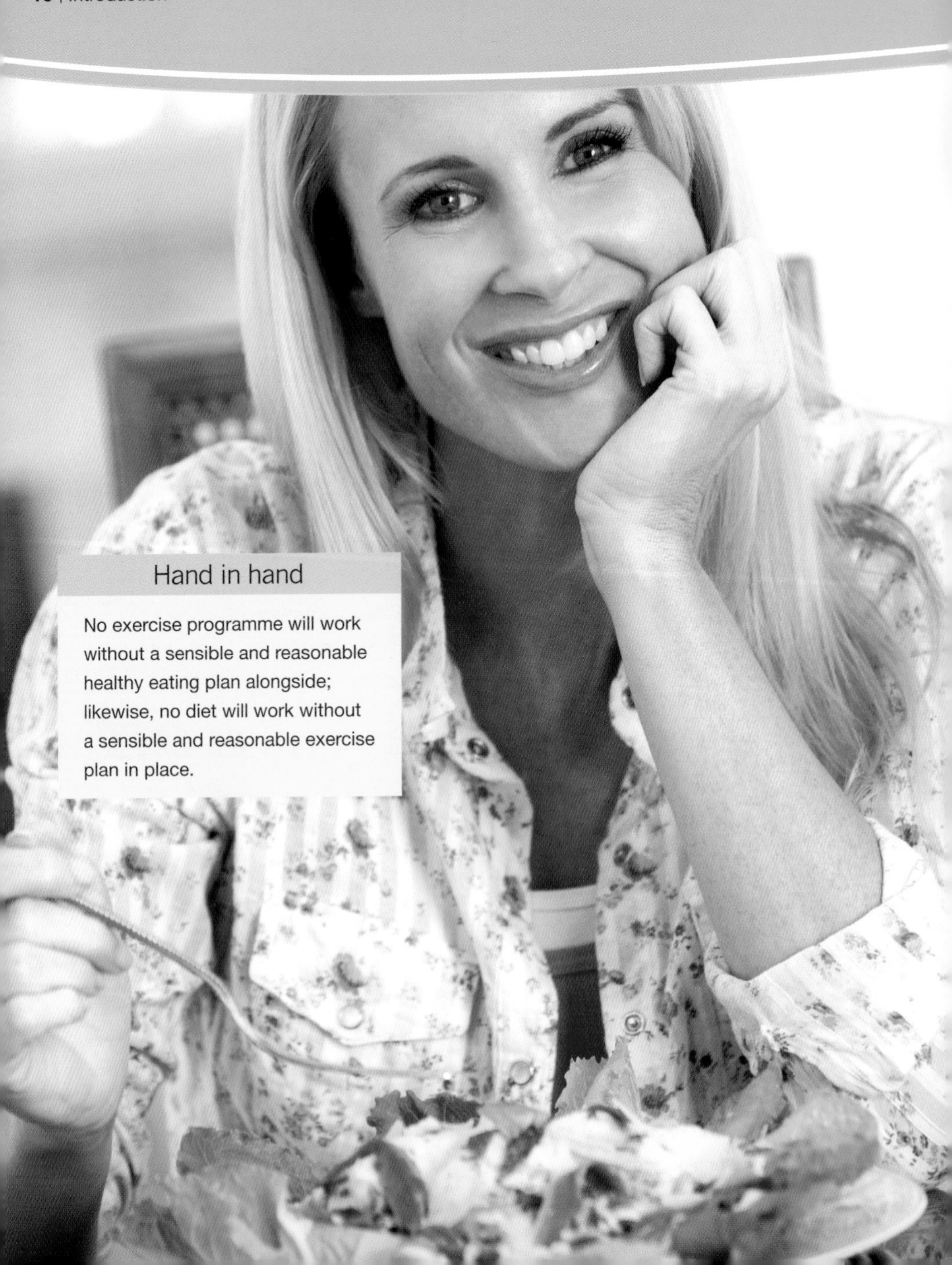

Hand in hand

No exercise programme will work without a sensible and reasonable healthy eating plan alongside; likewise, no diet will work without a sensible and reasonable exercise plan in place.

Fast Fit Works

Fast fitness isn't new. The amazing Roger Bannister, the first man recorded to run one mile in under four minutes in 1954, used the principle of fast bursts of intense exercise with recovery periods to build his body to peak condition.

There is a growing body of research from different studies around the world that shows that short, intense exercise patterns can lead to quicker weight loss and increased cardiovascular performance than more moderate exercise over a longer duration. Benefits of fast fitness can be seen quickly with a targeted, intense approach.

What's in a name?

There are many different programmes for fast-and-furious workouts and many variations. The principle behind all High Intensity Training (HIT) is the same: work hard for seconds or minutes, recover briefly and then repeat the exercise at high intensity.

The exercises in this book are fast fitness or high intensity exercises with recovery periods. They work on your cardiovascular performance and strength in minutes.

You can easily build these short workouts, which literally last minutes, into your busy week and you will feel and see the changes. Apart from swimming, you can do them pretty much anywhere and at any time.

But before you think this is all too good to be true and sit back – stop. Don't think that one minute of intense work will allow you to sit on the sofa eating chocolates for a week – it's not that easy! Although those minutes when you do exercise will be seriously hard, you need to remain relatively active for the rest of the week, and eat a healthy diet. Junk food will only impede the gains you make.

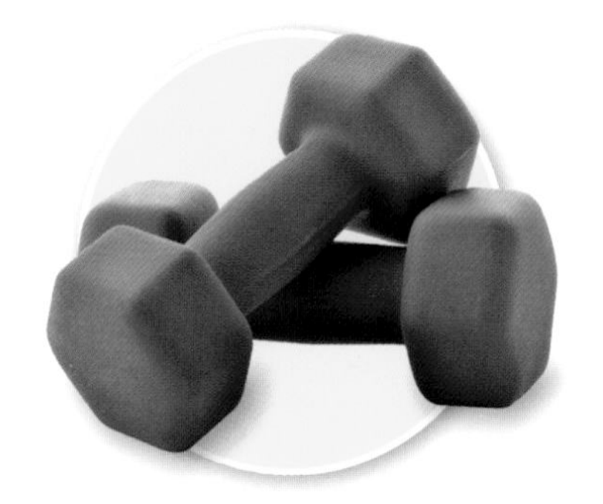

Who doesn't want to look good and fit into a great pair of jeans or look toned for the beach? Who isn't tempted by headlines promising that a new diet or special shoe will miraculously transform your body in five weeks with minimum effort? It would be great if it were that easy! The truth is that fit bodies are earned and maintained through the effort of regular exercise and healthy eating patterns over time.

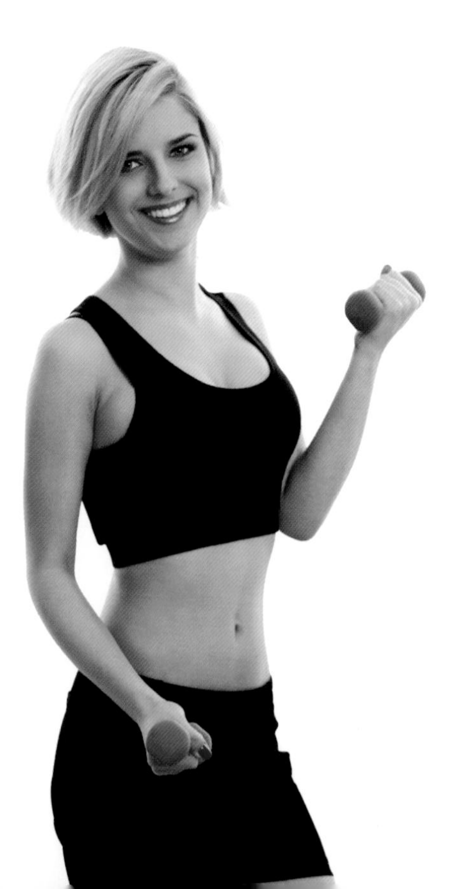

Feeling good

Fast fitness exercises are not easy; the programme is meant to be hard. It's going to make you feel like a sweaty, exhausted jelly afterwards. So why do we do it? The answer is that exercise makes us feel good, and of course it makes us look great. It also makes us healthier in both body and mind. Research shows that being fit lowers the risk of heart disease, type 2 diabetes and many other illnesses. You are likely to feel less stressed and sleep better. Your skin glows, your muscles are toned; your mood lifts and sex is better. All the arguments are in favour of getting fit – and fast.

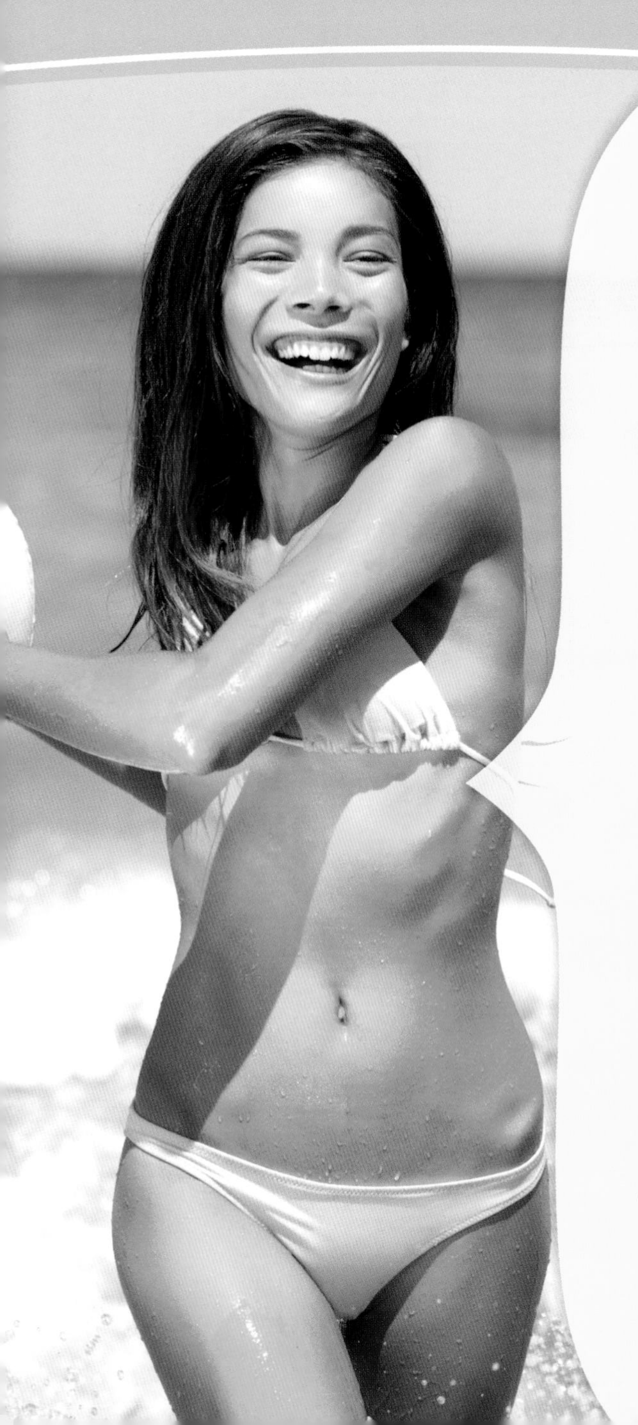

Aerobic training

Aerobic exercise is generally of moderate intensity over a longer duration than HIT. This type of exercise uses lots of oxygen that helps metabolise (break down) stored fat into energy. It raises your heart rate and makes you slightly breathless, keeping your heart, lungs and muscles healthy, and improves your fitness levels.

Anaerobic training

This training uses short blasts of explosive activity (one to three minutes). During this time the body is unable to supply enough oxygen quickly enough to the muscles to meet the energy expended. As a result, a waste product called lactic acid builds up. Oxygen is needed to remove the lactic acid – that's why you puff and pant after HIT, and why the recovery phase is so important.

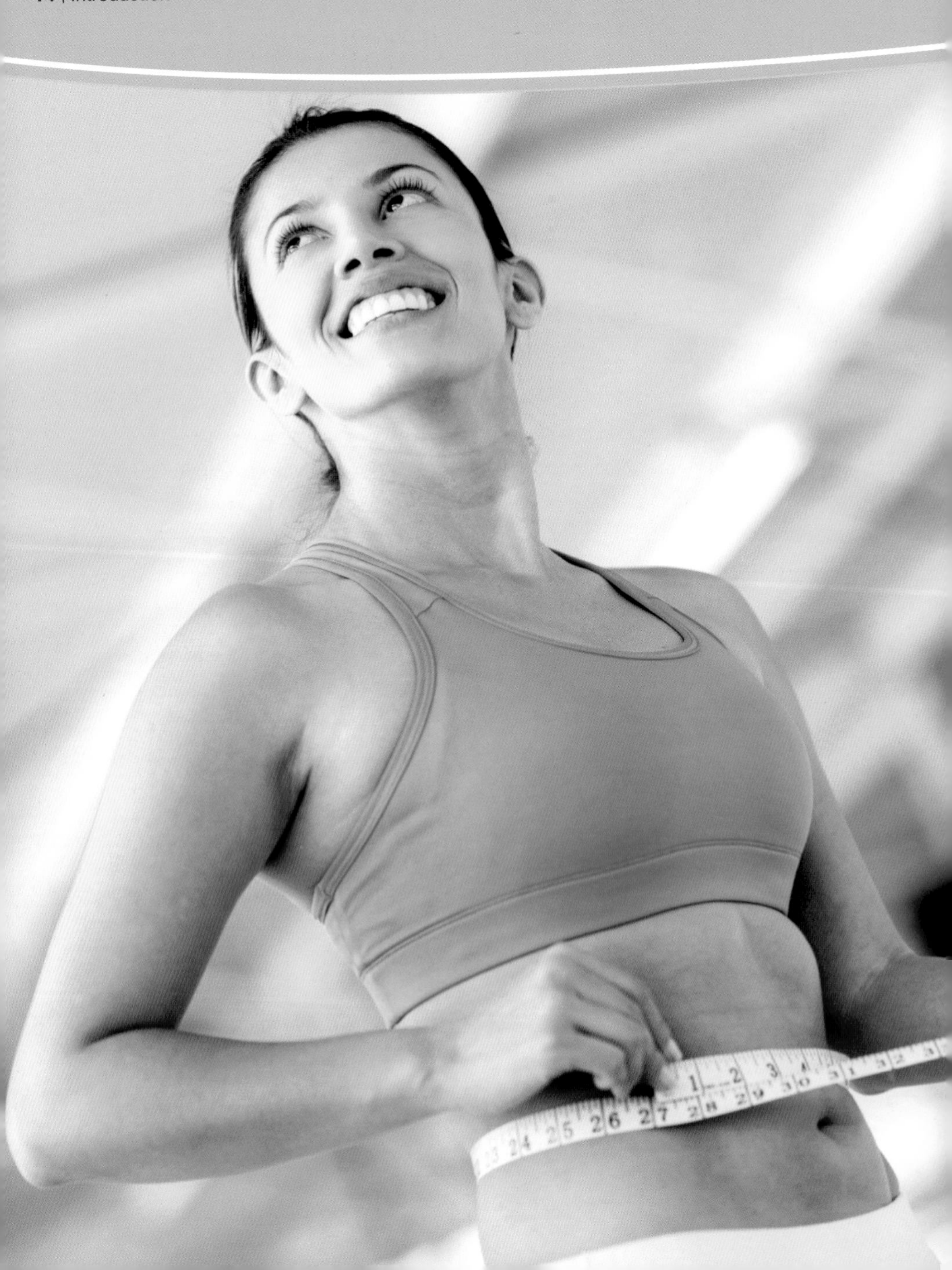

Science of Fast Fitness

Programmes promoting intense bursts of exercise have been marketed under many different names, but the principle behind the method is the same: several minutes of seriously hard exercise can help improve your fitness.

Periods of hard work are known as high intensity activity. Adding in rest periods (or intervals) increases the effects of the high intensity activity. These periods of rest allow your body to recover enough for you to repeat a minute or so of intense activity.

Working at high intensity helps weight loss as the body burns up fat more quickly than in sustained moderate exercise. The body's systems (respiratory and cardiovascular) work at such a pitch that more fat and calories are used to keep pace with the amount of energy used during HIT.

Because the body works flat out during HIT, it uses more calories to replace lost energy and continues to do so as the body's system slows.

Power packs

When you push to the max on your run, you are probably more aware of the burn in your thighs than the infinitesimally tiny power packs of your cells called mitochondria. When you work out at high intensity, the mitochondria in your muscle cells (and your heart, which is a large muscle) get to work transferring fat into energy.

Working to the max and then allowing the body to recover while doing gentle exercise has been shown to speed up the body's metabolic rate – the rate at which the body burns energy.

Health Aware

Fast fitness is quick but it is hard. In order to start this type of programme, you need to be in good health and already have a certain level of fitness.

It is a good idea to see your doctor before starting any intense exercise routine or programme, to check it is suitable. It is especially important to see a doctor before attempting any of the exercises in this book if you are unfit, suffer from health issues or are overweight.

In those instances, it may be more suitable to follow a less strenuous plan first to build up fitness and accommodate any particular health issues. When you reach a certain level of fitness, then you can pick up some of these more intense exercises or adapt them to suit your level of fitness. High intensity work is hard but it should not make you feel unwell. Listen to your body.

All of the exercises and routines in this book can be adapted in duration and intensity. You may be tempted to shorten your workout to five minutes instead of ten by leaving out the recovery period – don't. The recovery period allows your body to recover its strength to cope with the next burst of intensive work.

It is important not to work out at an intense level every day. Your body doesn't need it and won't react well to the relentless effort. Aim for about three times a week – after all, this exercise is meant to fit around your busy life, not the other way round. You can add the programme into your regular routine, for instance walking the dog or cycling to work, but don't overdo the high intensity exercise as it will put too much strain on your body.

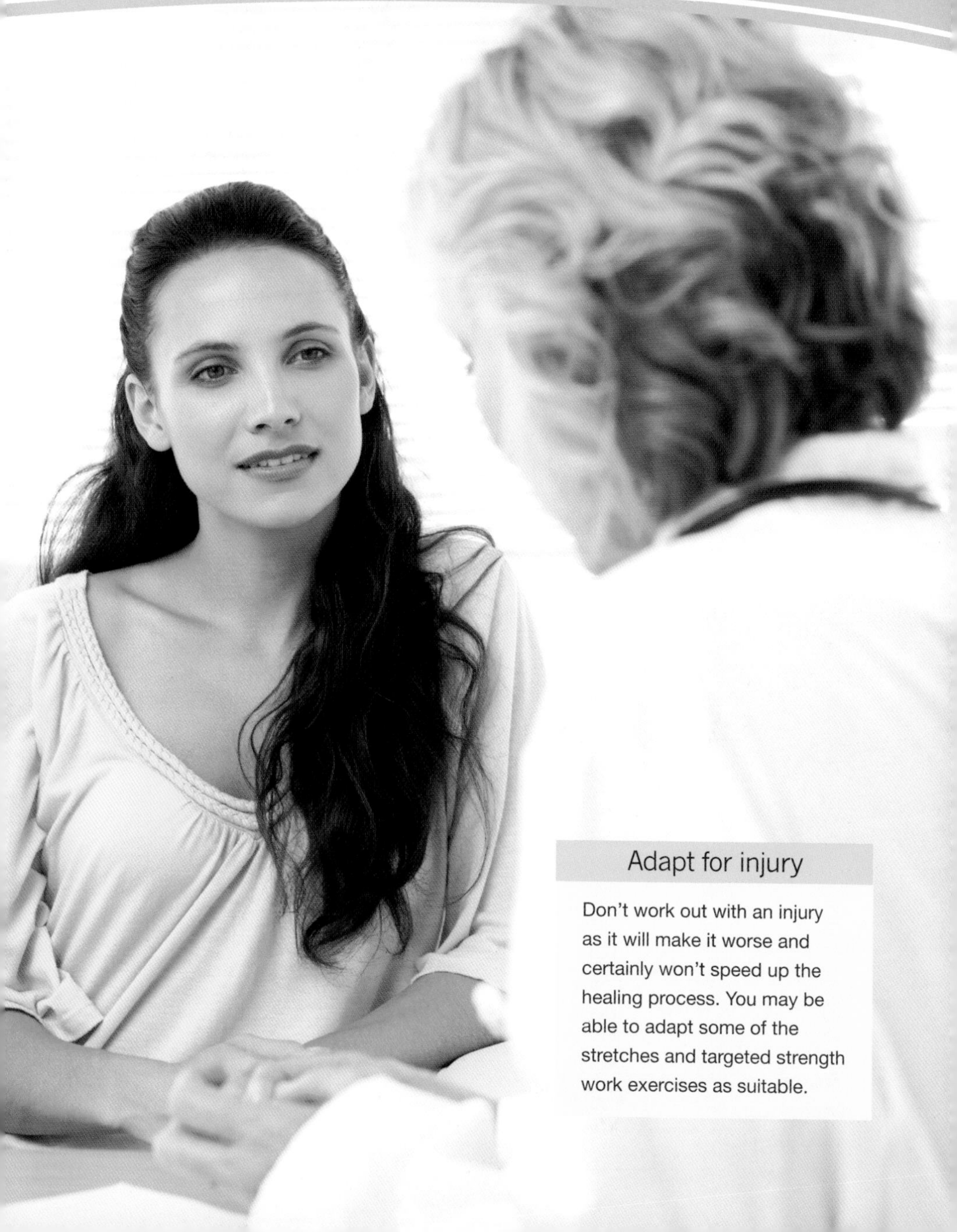

Adapt for injury

Don't work out with an injury as it will make it worse and certainly won't speed up the healing process. You may be able to adapt some of the stretches and targeted strength work exercises as suitable.

How to Use This Book

This book offers routines and exercises that are seriously hard, but last for minutes. You can pick and choose the exercises and how long you want to follow them, but it is all about hard work in a short space of time.

The exercises and routines in this book are grouped according to activity and effect:

- Running
- Cycling
- Swimming
- Circuits
- Weights

The routines combine intense exercise with recovery and aerobic and anaerobic fitness.

Each routine has a suggested duration for the warm-up, the exercise, the recovery and the number of repetitions. Ideally a warm-up should last five minutes, and the two-minute suggested warm-up is a minimum. These are all variable and adaptable to your level. Just make sure that you always include a recovery period. Do not work at a high intensity level for more than ten minutes at a time, three times a week.

Working at 85 per cent of your maximum heart rate is hard work. To begin with, aim for less intensity. Listen to your body, check your bpm (beats per minute, page 22) and build up to your peak. Use the diary sheets to record your progress (see pages 112–118).

As well as particular workouts, there is advice on how to make this training a natural and easy part of your life.

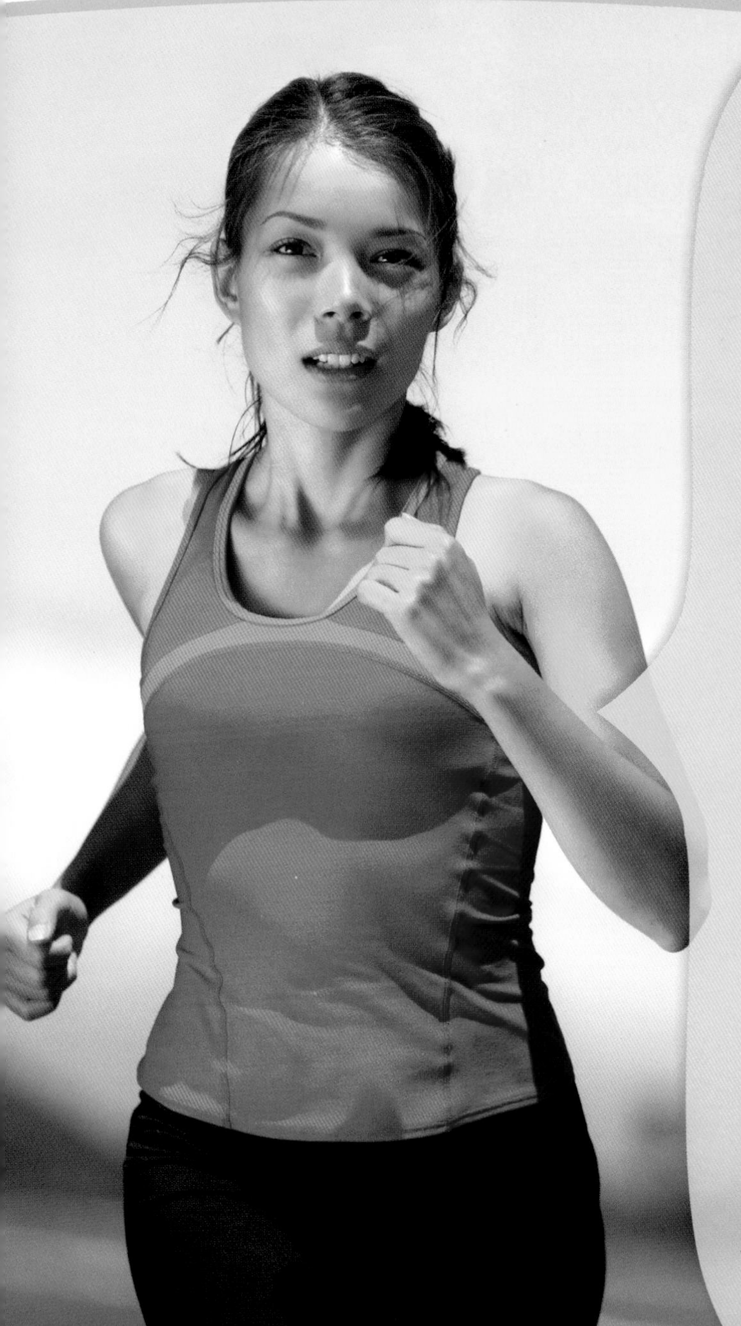

Do

- Do choose the exercises
- Do choose the rate at which you work to suit you and your abilities
- Do adapt the duration of each exercise
- Do choose the number of reps
- Do check with your doctor first if you are overweight, pregnant, unfit or suffer from health issues

Don't

- Don't miss the warm-up or cool down, or the recovery period
- Don't work at high intensity for more than ten minutes, three times a week

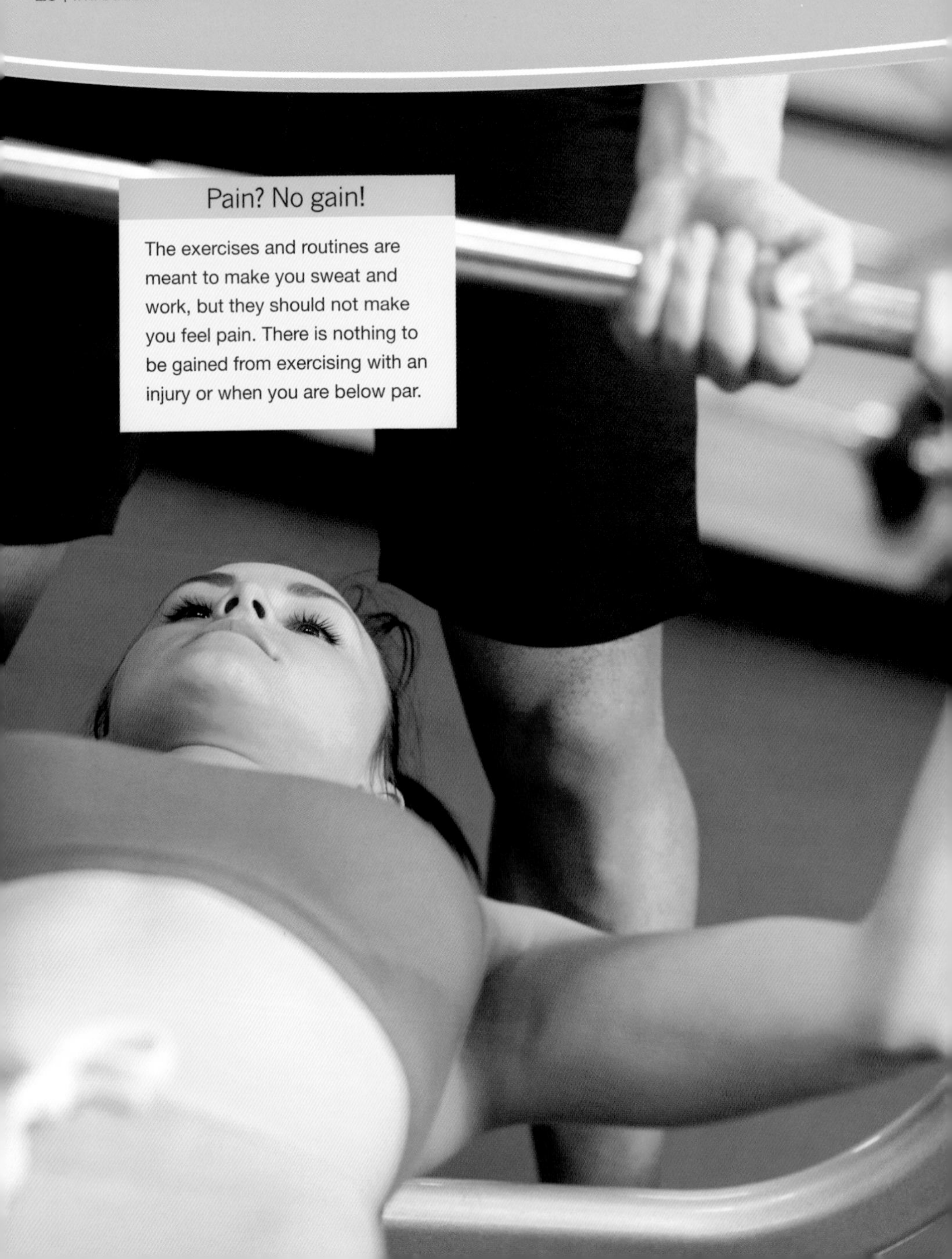

Pain? No gain!

The exercises and routines are meant to make you sweat and work, but they should not make you feel pain. There is nothing to be gained from exercising with an injury or when you are below par.

The exercises

The range of exercises in this book will work on the following key components of physical fitness.

Stamina

Sometimes this is referred to as cardiovascular fitness or muscular endurance. This allows you to work out for longer and involves exercise that works the heart and lungs, such as aerobics, running and cycling. This can be either aerobic or anaerobic. Cardiovascular training strengthens the heart (cardio) and the blood vessels (vascular) and helps improve your overall fitness.

Strength

This is being able to use muscles to apply force against resistance. Weight work will help with this.

Flexibility

This relates to your range of movement. Exercises for this keep your muscles stretchy – that's what allows you to touch your toes!

Hard enough?

You aren't working vigorously enough if you can talk to someone while you are working out, unless you are resting between reps.

Intensity check

Look up your maximum heartbeats per minute, bpm (see page 22). Check your pulse the moment you stop exercising, or invest in a heart monitor and work out the percentage. For example, if your bpm is the same as the maximum bpm, you are working at 100 per cent. Working at 60 per cent of your maximum is moderate intensity, and at 85 per cent is hard.

Rest periods

At the start, aim for a ratio of 1:3, exercise to recovery. As your fitness increases, you can decrease the amount of recovery and increase the percentage at which your heart rate is working. Do not work at a high intensity for more than 10 minutes without a recovery period.

Fast Fit Ready

Most adults have a resting heart rate of 60–100 beats per minute. The fitter you are, the lower your resting heart rate is likely to be. For example, athletes may have a resting heart rate of 40–60 bpm or lower. When you exercise hard, your heart rate will increase. Intense exercise can increase your heart rate up to 85 per cent of its capacity. Your bpm gives you an indication of the intensity of your workout, but it's not always easy to take it mid-run! A heart rate monitor can check your bpm for you. If you prefer, check it by taking your pulse.

On the pulse

Find the pulse in your wrist:

- Hold out one of your hands with your palm facing upwards and your elbow slightly bent

- Press the index and middle finger of your other hand on the inside of your wrist, below your thumb, until you can feel your pulse

- Count the number of beats in 60 seconds (or 30 x 2). The number of beats is your heart rate

What max?

There are several ways to work out your maximum heart rate. You can do this in a gym on a treadmill with specific equipment. Alternatively, you can use a formula which, although not exact because it is very general, can give you an idea. The maximum heart rate is 220 bpm minus your age, so if you are 28 it will be 192, and if you are 35 it will be 185. So if you are 28 and working at 70 per cent, your heart rate will be around 134 bpm, and if you are 35 it will be around 129 bpm. As a guide, working at 60–65 per cent of your maximum is low intensity, and working at 75–85 per cent of your maximum is high intensity.

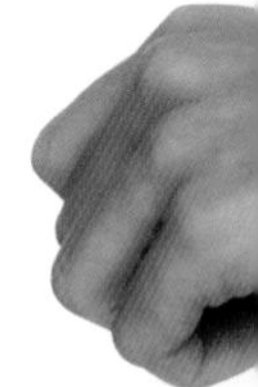

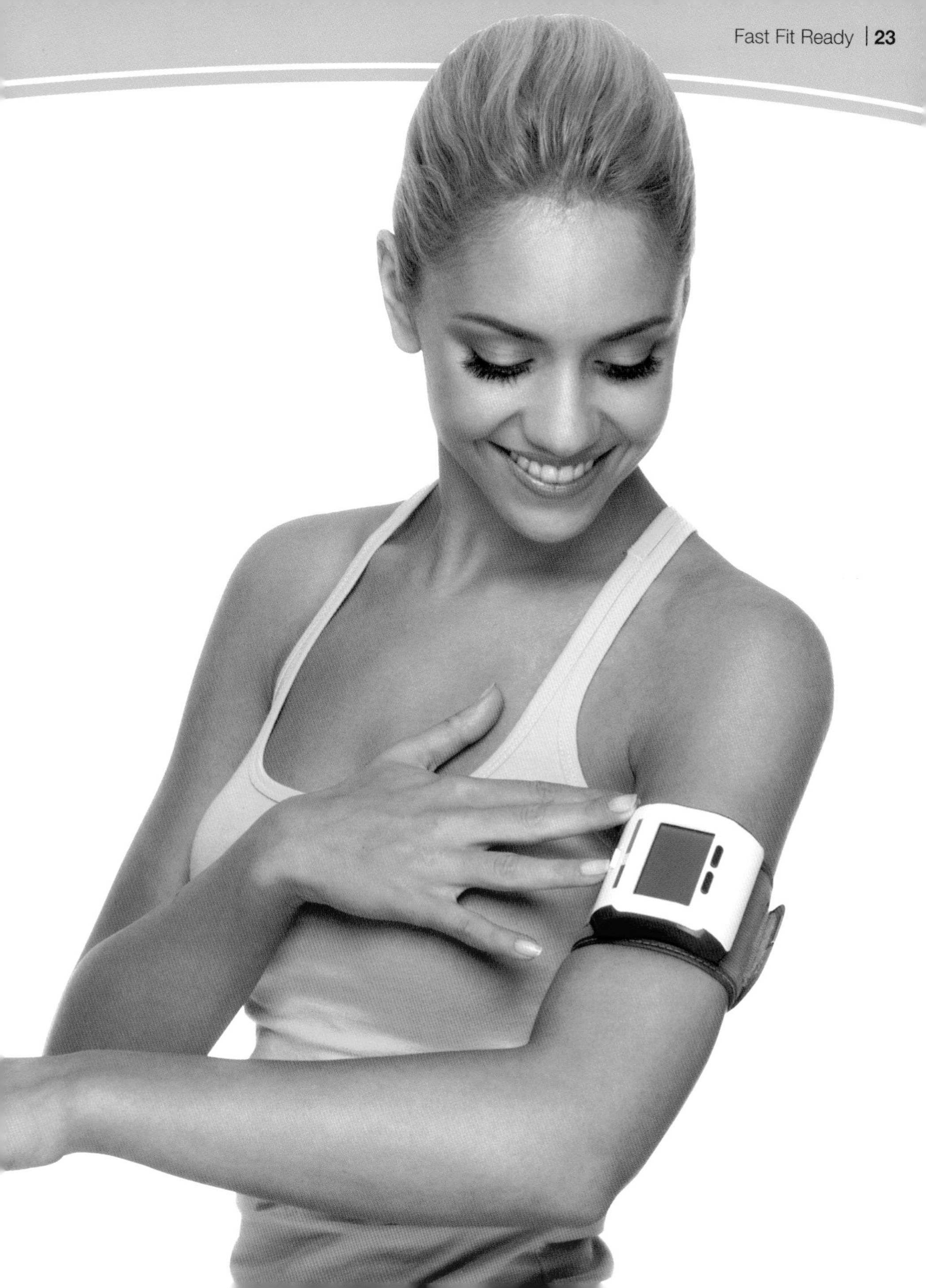

Measure

Before you start, you need to measure your fitness, and waist! Once you have a measure of your original fitness levels, you can check your progress on a weekly or fortnightly basis.

Jump

To measure your speed and strength, or power, jump! Stand against a wall with your hands above your head. Ask someone to mark lightly on the wall where your fingertips reach. Turn sideways to the wall, and jump as high as you can with your fingers outstretched. Record the distance between the two marks. After a couple of weeks of training, repeat.

Body Mass Index

Body Mass Index (BMI) is another way to measure your progress. This is an estimate of body composition. To work out your BMI, divide your weight (kilograms) by height (metres). Divide the answer by your height to get your BMI.

Testing!

Only do this fitness test if you are reasonably fit and do not have a history of medical problems. You will need a stopwatch and two cones or markers.

1. Put the cones 20 metres apart. See how many shuttle runs (between the cones) you can do in one minute. Run right to the cones.

2. Have one minute's rest and then try and beat that score.

3. Have another one minute rest and try again.

4. Continue this until you have done it five times. Note down your results and work out how many runs you did in the five minutes of shuttles.

5. See if you can beat the total.

6. Check your bpm (see page 22) immediately after one minute's sprint to see what your heart rate is. This will give you an indication of your bpm when you are working to about 85 per cent of your maximum capacity.

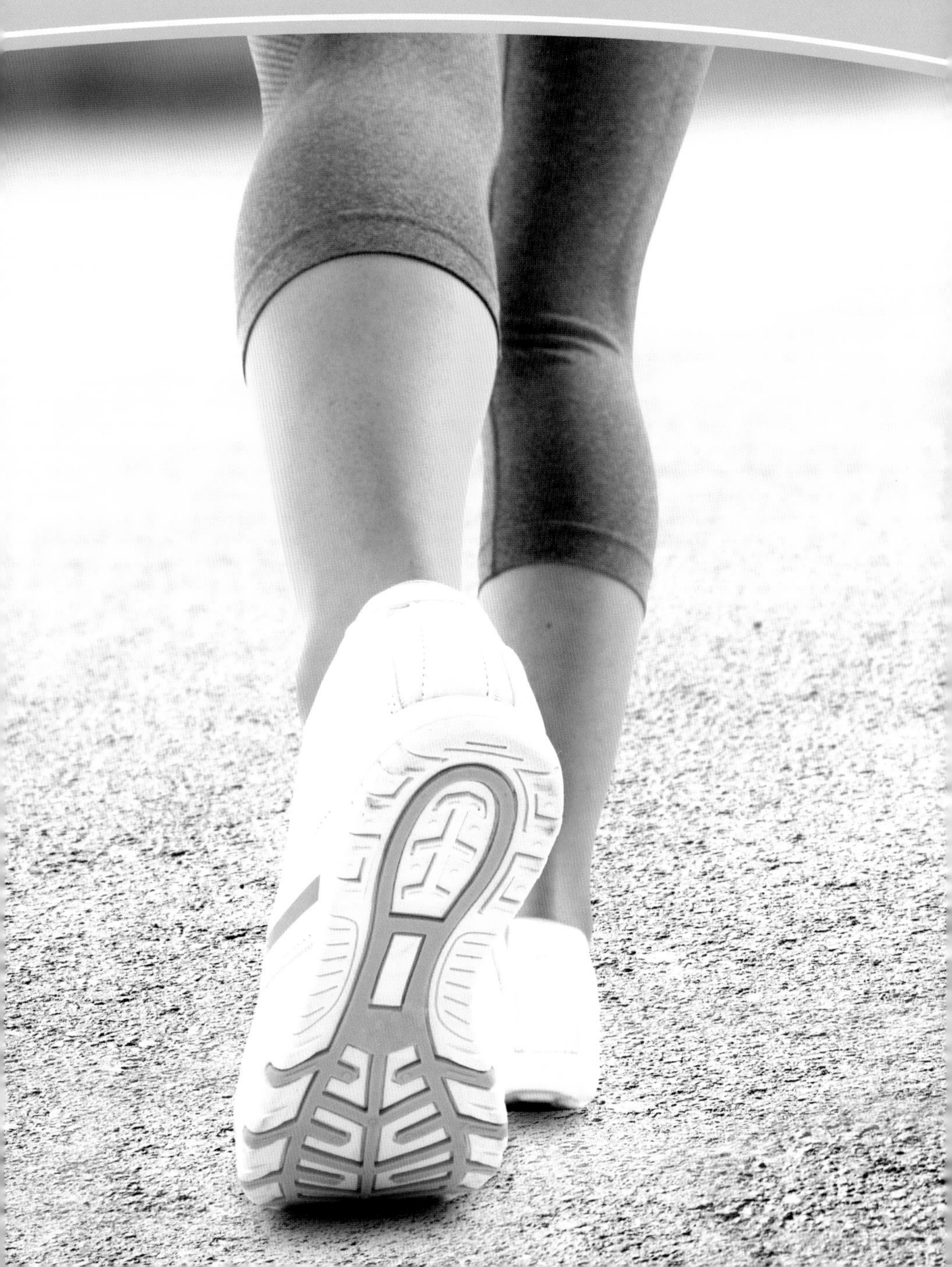

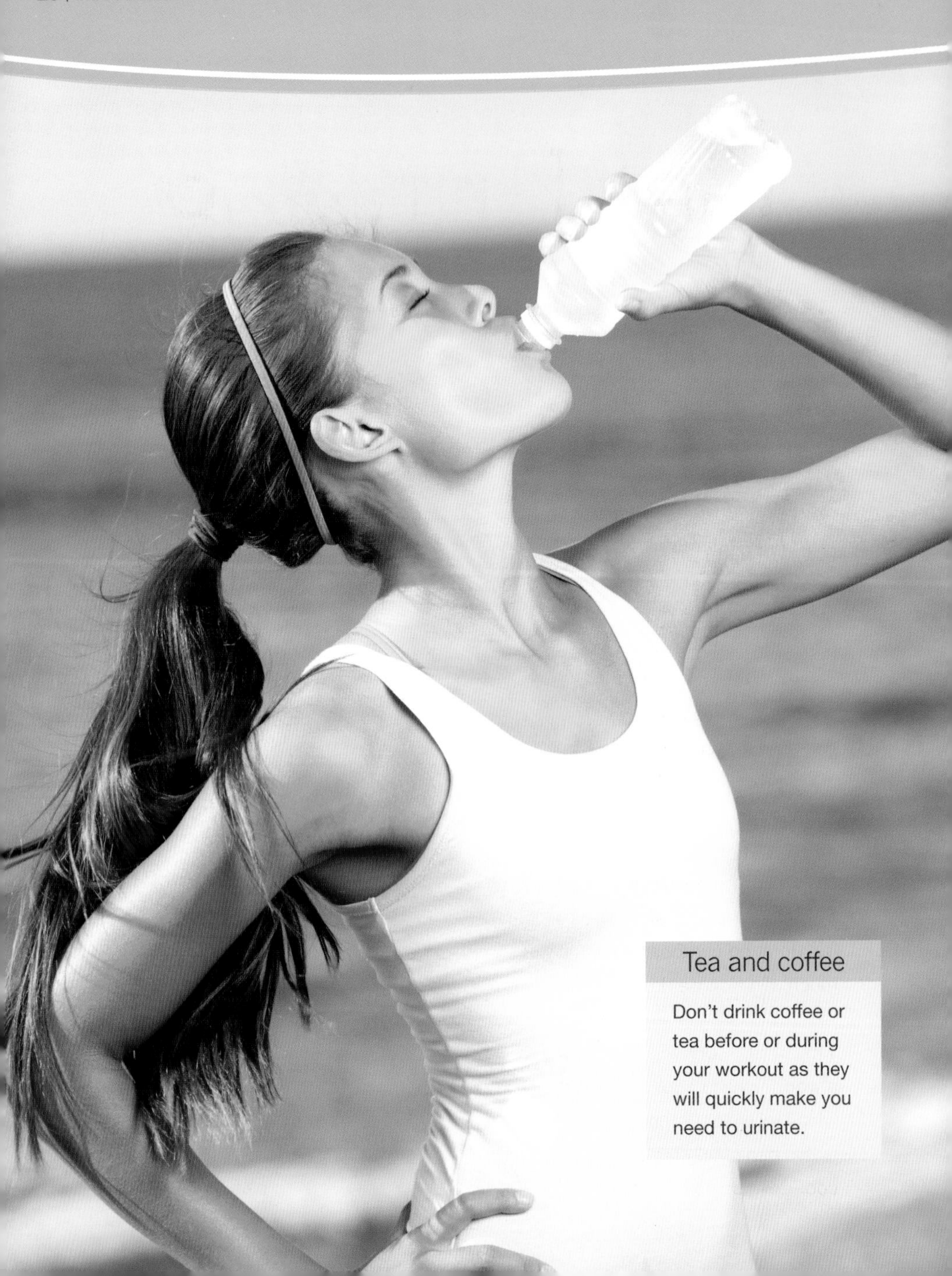

Tea and coffee

Don't drink coffee or tea before or during your workout as they will quickly make you need to urinate.

Get Drinking

The key to successful workouts is to make sure you are hydrated (have enough fluid in your body) before you start exercising, during and after you exercise.

If you are dehydrated before you start, your temperature will rise quickly and your heart will have to work very hard. This is dangerous. If your urine is dark coloured, it is a sign that you are dehydrated. You need to drink slowly but plenty at least four hours before you start exercising to make sure you are hydrated enough to exercise.

When you exercise hard you will sweat, so you need to replace the lost fluids. Drink plenty afterwards as well but don't go overboard; drinking too much can also be dangerous.

Time is short but you must always do a warm-up and cool-down, both of which include stretches. Each section in this book includes warm-ups and cool-downs.

Warm up

Prepare your body for what is about to come. Get your heart pumping and blood flowing around your body by light jogging, gentle cycling or a slow lap of the pool.

Rest

The rest or recovery periods in the routines are part of the high intensity pattern. Unless you allow your body to rest, you won't be able to continue your next set or rep at high intensity. These periods are not optional!

Cool down

Cooling down allows your body to adjust from high intensity activity to becoming sedentary. If you don't cool down you might feel lightheaded or dizzy, as all the blood pumping around your body during your workout suddenly drops to your lower limbs.

Fast Fitness Choices

Take your pick when it comes to fast exercises! From running to swimming, circuits to cycles, the choice is yours. For maximum benefit, mix and match so that your body is pushed and stretched and you work a wide range of muscles.

Running

This is hard on your knees but great for the heart. It's excellent aerobic exercise over a longer distance and anaerobic when sprinting.

Cycling

For this you need a bicycle (or a gym with a bike). It's great exercise for toning thighs and bums.

Swimming

An excellent all-over workout, but you do need a pool! It's not advisable to practice intense swimming exercises in the sea or rivers because of unpredictable currents and general safety concerns.

Circuits

Take it to the park, do it at home – circuits keep it lively and interesting. Varying your exercises in this way helps you work all parts of your body.

Weights

There's no need to worry that you will look like a body builder. You won't unless you work very hard to achieve that look. Sensible and moderate use of weights provides an excellent strength workout. You don't even need to do this in the gym!

Fun fit

Dancing, bouncing on a trampoline – both can be done at a high intensity level or incorporated into your weekly training programme.

Fast walk

You can even do it in your work wear!

Quick fix for bums and tums

This is great when you have a spare five minutes and want to work on a particular problem area.

Mix it up

If you keep your fast fitness routines varied it will help to maintain your interest. By mixing up your activities, your body is also more likely to respond quickly to each work out.

Stretches

You might think these are a lightweight version of exercise, but done properly and with real effort, they are an important way of keeping you supple and toned. If you are exercising for fast-and-furious intervals, do include stretches in your workout, otherwise your muscles can become shorter and less elastic, resulting in stiffness and an increased risk of injury.

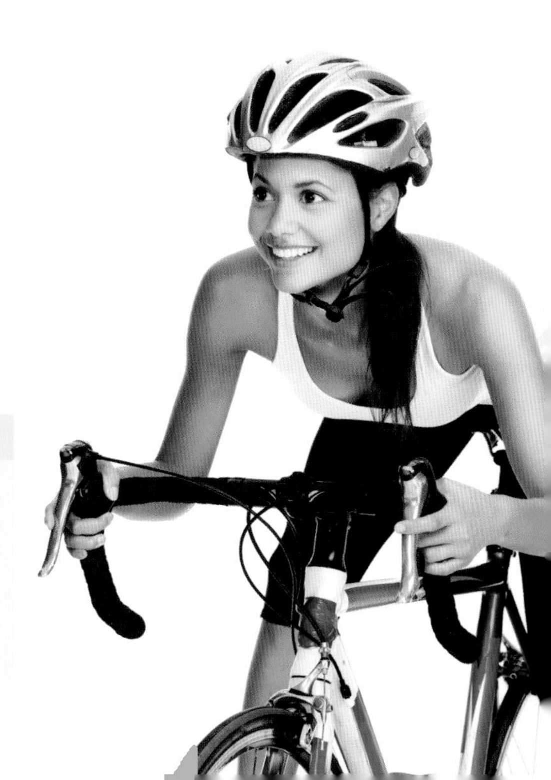

Running

The beauty of running is that you can take off wherever you are! All you need is a good pair of trainers.

Warm up

A warm-up is essential if you are going to run at high intensity. Obviously, it's not a good idea to go from sitting down at your desk for two hours to a crazily fast sprint without warming up! Your muscles won't like it. To warm up:

- Raise your arms and circle them clockwise and anticlockwise (it's not just your legs that are involved in running). Roll your shoulders back and forth to relax them
- Swivel your hips in circles and gently swivel your torso
- Lightly run on the spot for approximately 20 seconds

See also the stretches on page 37.

The workout

A: Total time 7 minutes 20 seconds

2 minute warm-up

20 seconds run (high intensity)

80 seconds recovery

Repeat 2 times

2 minute cool-down and stretch out

To begin with, aim to work at 75 per cent of your maximum. Build up gradually.

You'll be surprised at first how long 20 seconds feels when working hard.

Happy hormones

Running, like other cardiovascular exercise, releases hormones called endorphins. These are responsible for making us feel happy. So get moving!

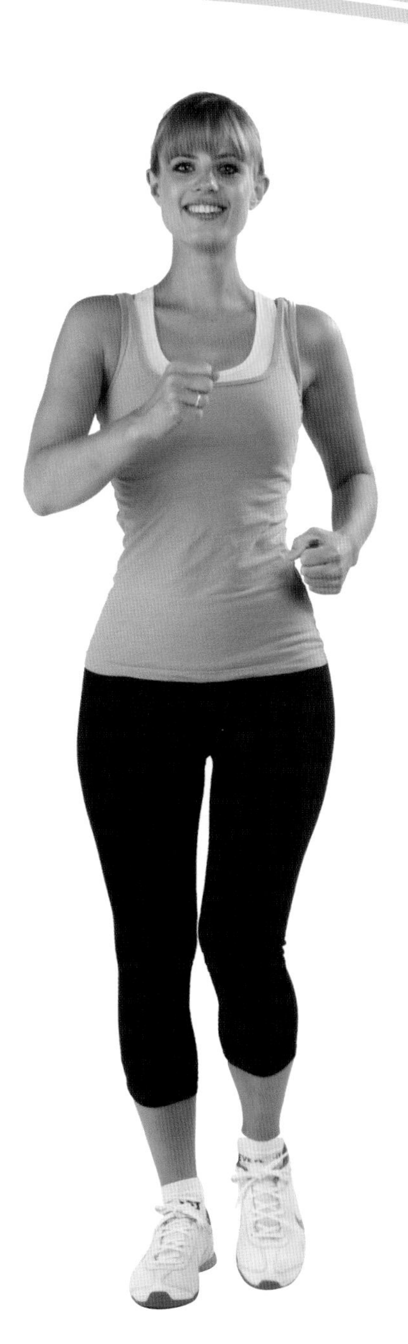

B: Total time 8 minutes 30 seconds

2 minute warm-up

30 seconds run

60 seconds recovery

Repeat 3 times

2 minute cool-down and stretch out

Try this for a week (maximum three times). If you run in the same place each time, see if you run further in the same time (use markers such as trees or lampposts).

During your recovery continue to move your legs by gentle jogging or walking – this will keep blood flowing around them and help get rid of waste products that built up when you sprint.

C: Total time 9 minutes

2 minute warm-up

40 seconds run

60 seconds recovery

Repeat 3 times

2 minute cool-down and stretch out

Remember, at high intensity you will feel shaky with the effort.

D: Total time 17 minutes

2 minute warm-up

60 seconds run

2 minutes recovery

Start with four reps (repetitions); gradually aim to build up to 10 reps

3 minute cool-down and stretch out

Repeat the above, and aim to work at 80 per cent of your maximum intensity. Don't forget your recovery periods – they are crucial.

And even more! (Advanced)

Warm-up

3 minutes run

3 minutes recovery

Repeat 6 times

5 minute cool-down and stretch out

Variations
(10–20 minutes, moderate)
For a less intense workout, run fast (but not at your maximum) for one minute; rest for one minute, and then repeat this 10 or 20 times.

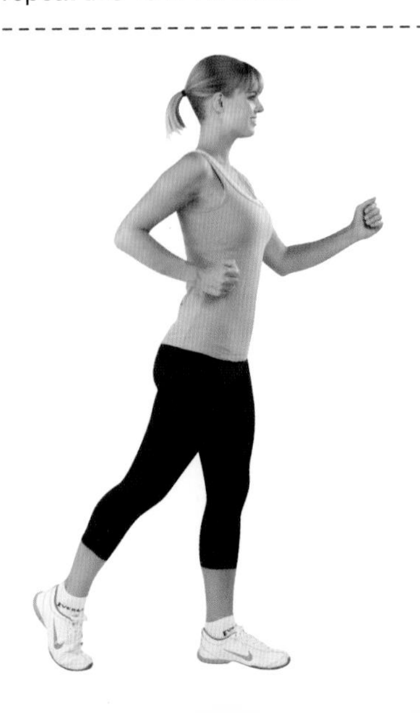

Your technique

You've probably run to catch the bus, missing it just as the driver knowingly closes the door while you pant to the finish line – but you probably weren't thinking of your technique then! Now is the time to perfect an effective and comfortable style so that you run smoothly – yes, even when you are sprinting.

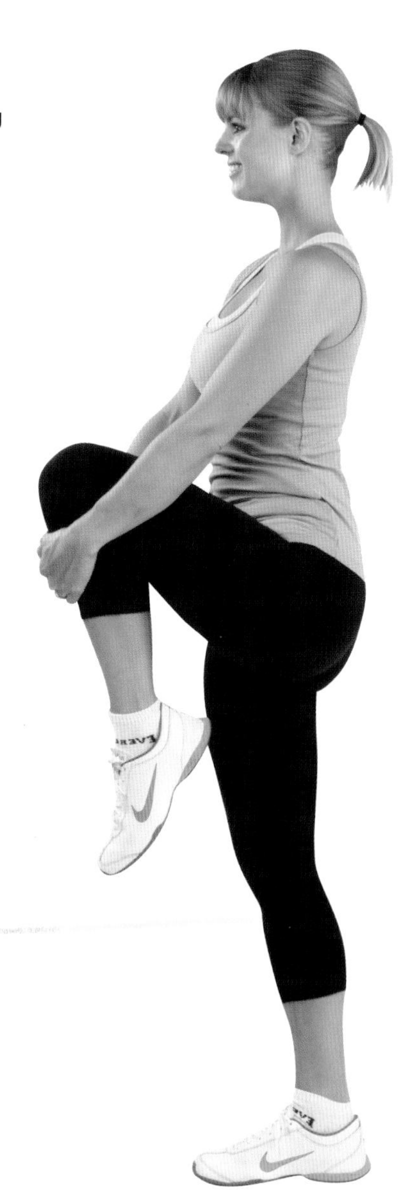

- Once you have accelerated, lift your torso and try not to lean forward – it won't make you go faster
- Hold your head high and keep your gaze naturally ahead
- Keep your shoulders down and not tucked up into your neck – the temptation on a sprint is to tense up, but you actually want the flow of your movement to enhance your speed
- Let your arms work too – keep your elbows at a right angle, and swing your hands up to shoulder height and then back down by your hips
- Imagine your legs circling from your hips. When you sprint, lift your knees high to help give you power and speed. Aim to strike the ground lightly with the ball of your foot

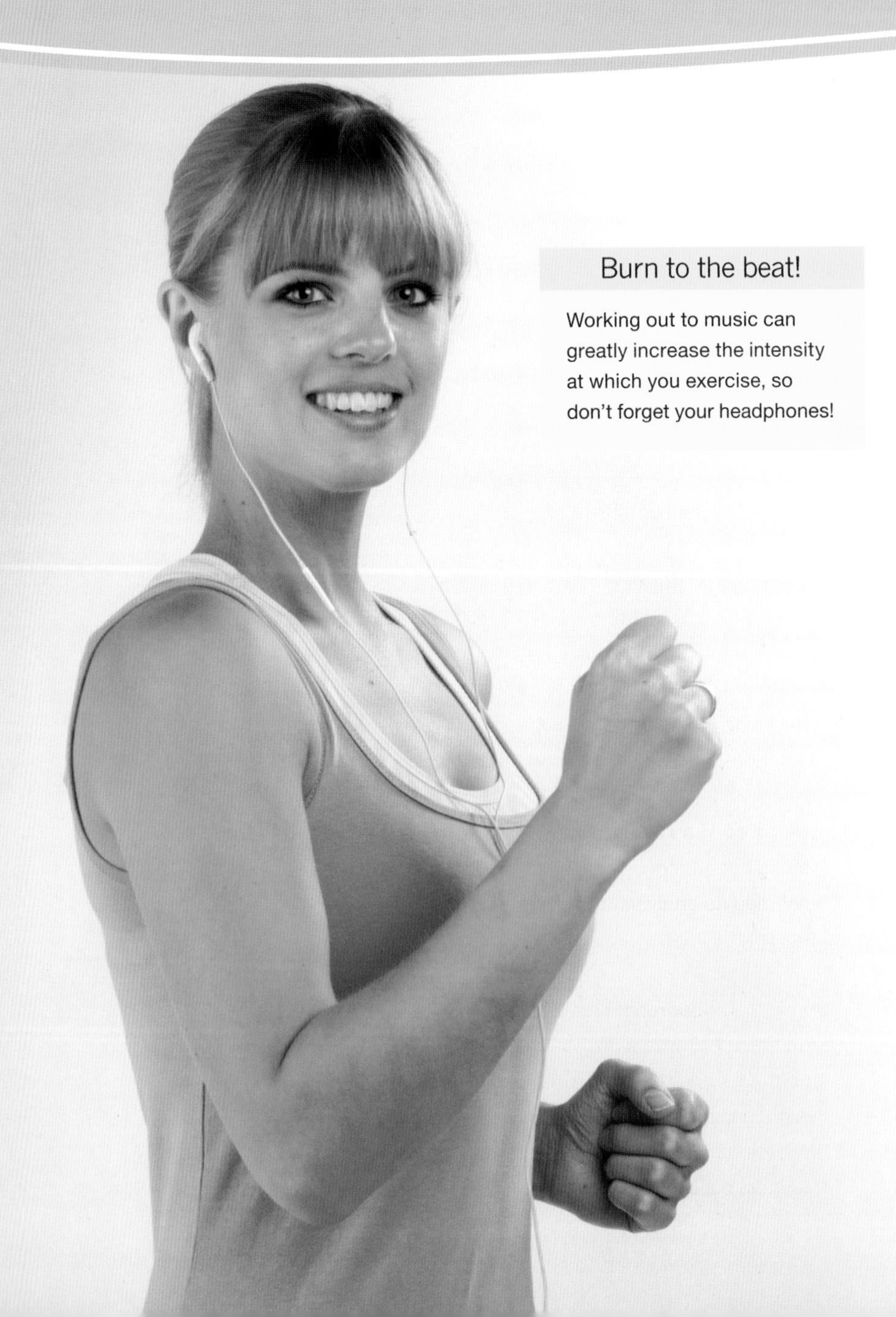

Burn to the beat!

Working out to music can greatly increase the intensity at which you exercise, so don't forget your headphones!

On the treadmill

Some people love them, and others loathe them. Treadmills don't give you fresh air (or a lungful of pollution, depending on where you are running!) but they can be set directly to your challenge: simply get on, work out, get off and rest. And it doesn't rain on a treadmill...

You need to feel confident adjusting the speed on a treadmill – you don't want to hurtle backwards in a heap because you have literally moved from standstill to sprint.

There's no wind resistance on a treadmill – running flat on a treadmill is easier than running on the flat in the open air, so you need to adjust the setting accordingly. This is generally accepted as equivalent to a one per cent incline on the treadmill setting.

As with outdoor running, warm up and then start with a one-minute sprint, rest and repeat four times. Next time, increase the speed and then the duration. As with all these routines, build up slowly.

Power music

Some people find music a great motivator for distance running. Choose something with a fast beat for your sprints.

A: Total time 16 minutes

2 minute warm-up

1 minute run at 65 per cent of max

1 minute recovery

Repeat 6 times

2 minute cool-down and stretch out

B: Total time 11 minutes 30 seconds (Advanced)

2 minute warm-up

30 seconds run at 85 per cent of max

1 minute recovery

Repeat 5 times

2 minute cool-down and stretch out

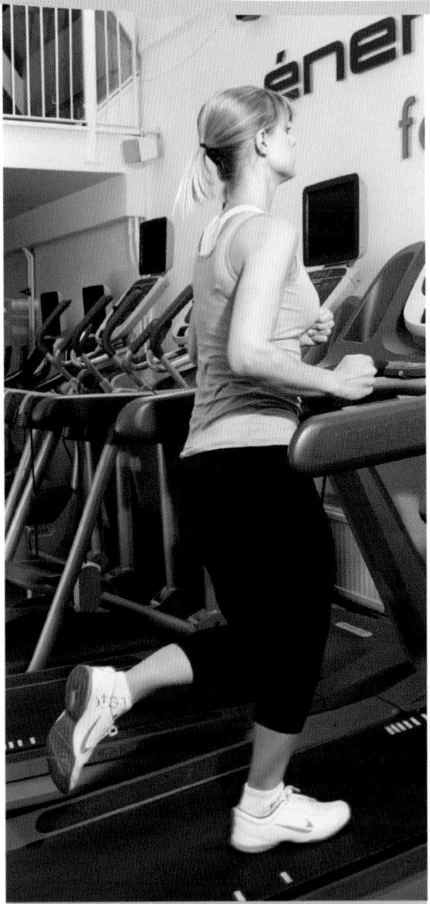

Uphill

Ok, now it's time to try running uphill. Be warned – this is hard. Walk down afterwards as part of your cool down. Olympic Champion Sebastian Coe, whose trainer included lots of uphill runs, always drove him back down to avoid the strain on his joints of running downhill.

Workout

Repeat the exercises on page 35, but going uphill.

Cool it

Vary your cool down – you don't just have to run in a straight line. After your HIT sprint, run backwards (but not on a busy road, hill or anywhere you are likely to crash into something). It is best to do this if you are with a running mate. It's great for co-ordination and balance, and you won't be tempted to do it at speed.

Safe exercise

Running outdoors is more challenging in terms of personal safety than running on a treadmill in the gym. When running in the dark, make sure you are easily visible by wearing a reflective strip or top. It is also safer to run with a friend or running group.

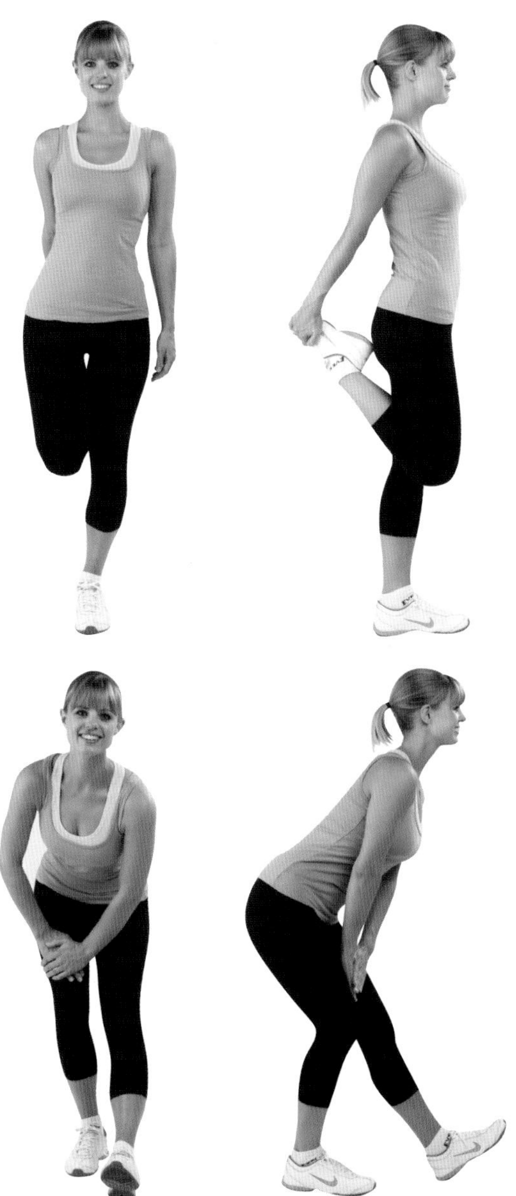

Stretch

After your run (whatever the intensity or duration), stretch your muscles out to prevent them from seizing up. Key stretches:

- Stretch your thigh as you bring your heel to your buttock and hold it for ten seconds. Repeat on the other leg
- Stretch your hamstring. Bend one leg and extend the other leg in front of you with your heel on the ground but the rest of the foot raised. Gently lean over the extended leg and feel the stretch. Repeat on the other side
- Stretch your calf. Place both hands against a wall. Extend one leg backwards. Keep it straight with your foot flat on the floor. Step your other leg forwards with your foot flat and bend at the knee. Lean into the wall and stretch the calf of your extended back leg. Repeat on the other side

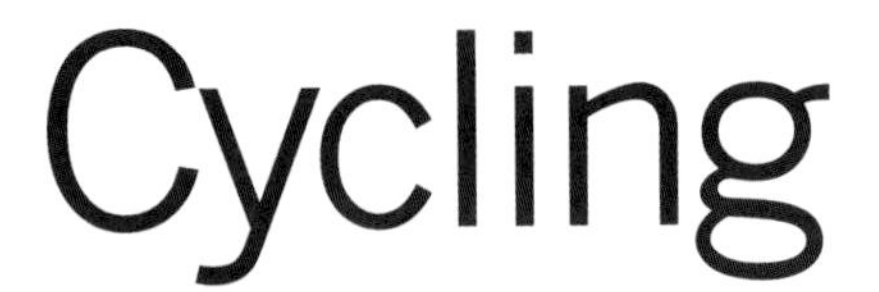

Cycling

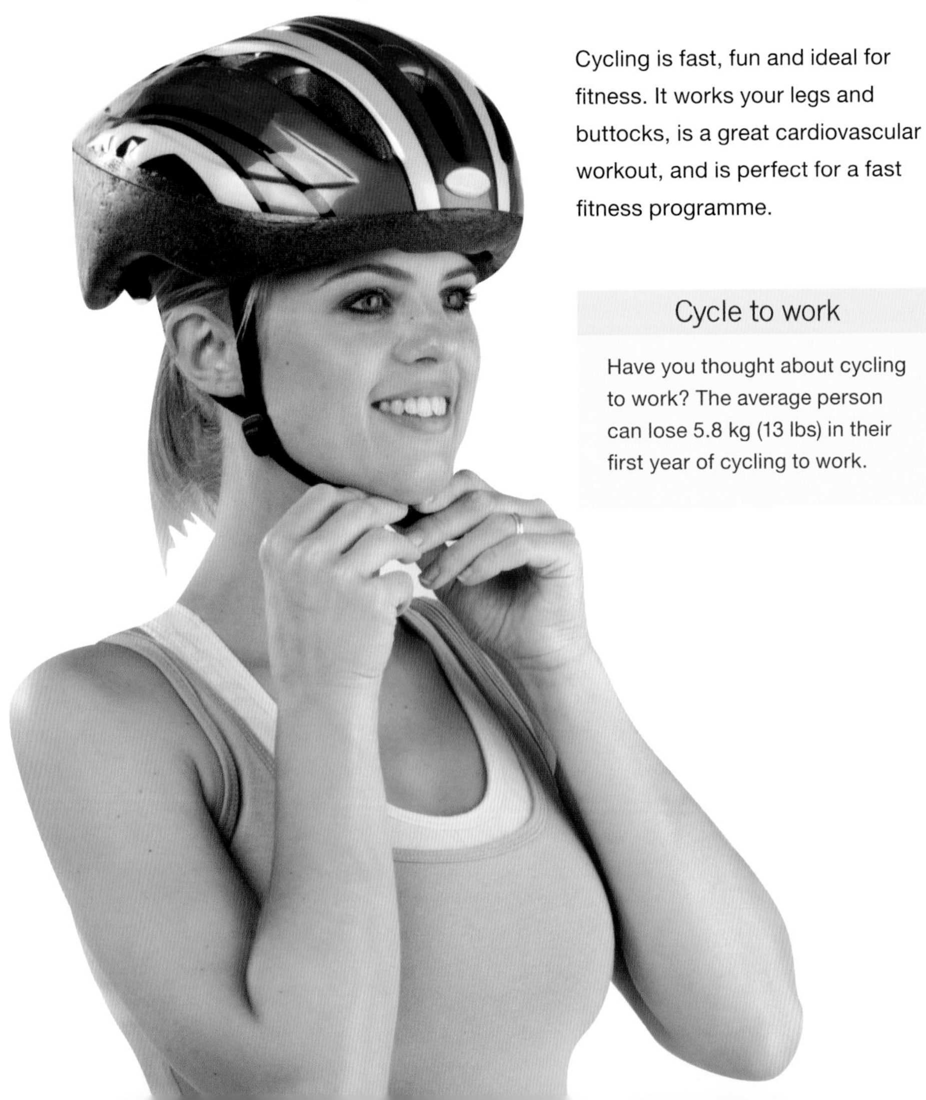

Cycling is fast, fun and ideal for fitness. It works your legs and buttocks, is a great cardiovascular workout, and is perfect for a fast fitness programme.

Cycle to work

Have you thought about cycling to work? The average person can lose 5.8 kg (13 lbs) in their first year of cycling to work.

Bike fit

It sounds obvious but easy to overlook – check your bike is fit for use before you start. The brakes must be in good condition, as you will be using pedal power to move at speed.

As with using any piece of equipment, make sure it fits your size. Check the saddle height by putting the balls of your feet on the pedals. Turn the pedal until it is at the bottom of the pedal stroke: in this position your knee should be slightly bent. Your leg is neither cramped nor overstretched.

Where's your foot?

Try to cycle with the balls of your feet on the pedals and with your feet facing straight forwards. It sounds obvious, but make sure your laces are tucked away so that they don't get caught in the spokes as you cycle.

Body conscious

Your torso should be leaning forwards, and your elbows should be bent.

Safety

As you will be cycling fast, wear a helmet. It's an important piece of kit and will keep you safe. If you are pedalling at high speed, you must make sure that the track is clear and safe. It is not safe to try out a burst of intense speed on a busy road.

Make sure the terrain is suitable for speed. It's one thing to pedal over bumpy ground when at leisure, but quite another when you are focused on using all your energy for maximum effort. Watch out for dogs (and their walkers) stepping out into your path.

Warm up

As well as doing some hamstring and calf stretches (see page 37), stretch out your back. Put your feet shoulder distance apart and lean forward, holding onto your bike with your hands shoulder-width apart. Push your chest downwards, keeping your back straight. You might feel a light stretch in the back of your legs, but will feel more of a stretch in your upper back.

Cycle it up

Spend at least five minutes riding at a gentle and then moderate pace before starting these workouts.

A: Total time 7 minutes 20 seconds

2 minute warm-up

20 seconds cycle (high intensity)

80 seconds recovery

Repeat 2 times

2 minute cool-down and stretch out

At first, aim to work at 70–75 per cent of your maximum. Build up gradually.

B: Total time 8 minutes 30 seconds

2 minute warm-up

30 seconds cycle (high intensity)

60 seconds recovery

Repeat 3 times

2 minute cool-down and stretch out

C: Total time 9 minutes

2 minute warm-up

40 seconds cycle (high intensity)

60 seconds recovery

Repeat 3 times

2 minute cool-down and stretch out

D: Total time 17 minutes

2 minute warm-up

60 seconds cycle (high intensity)

2 minutes recovery

Start with 4 reps; aim to build up to 8 reps (advanced)

3 minute cool-down and stretch out

Technique

- Keep your abdominal muscles working and tight
- Don't let your back sag down between your shoulders and hips

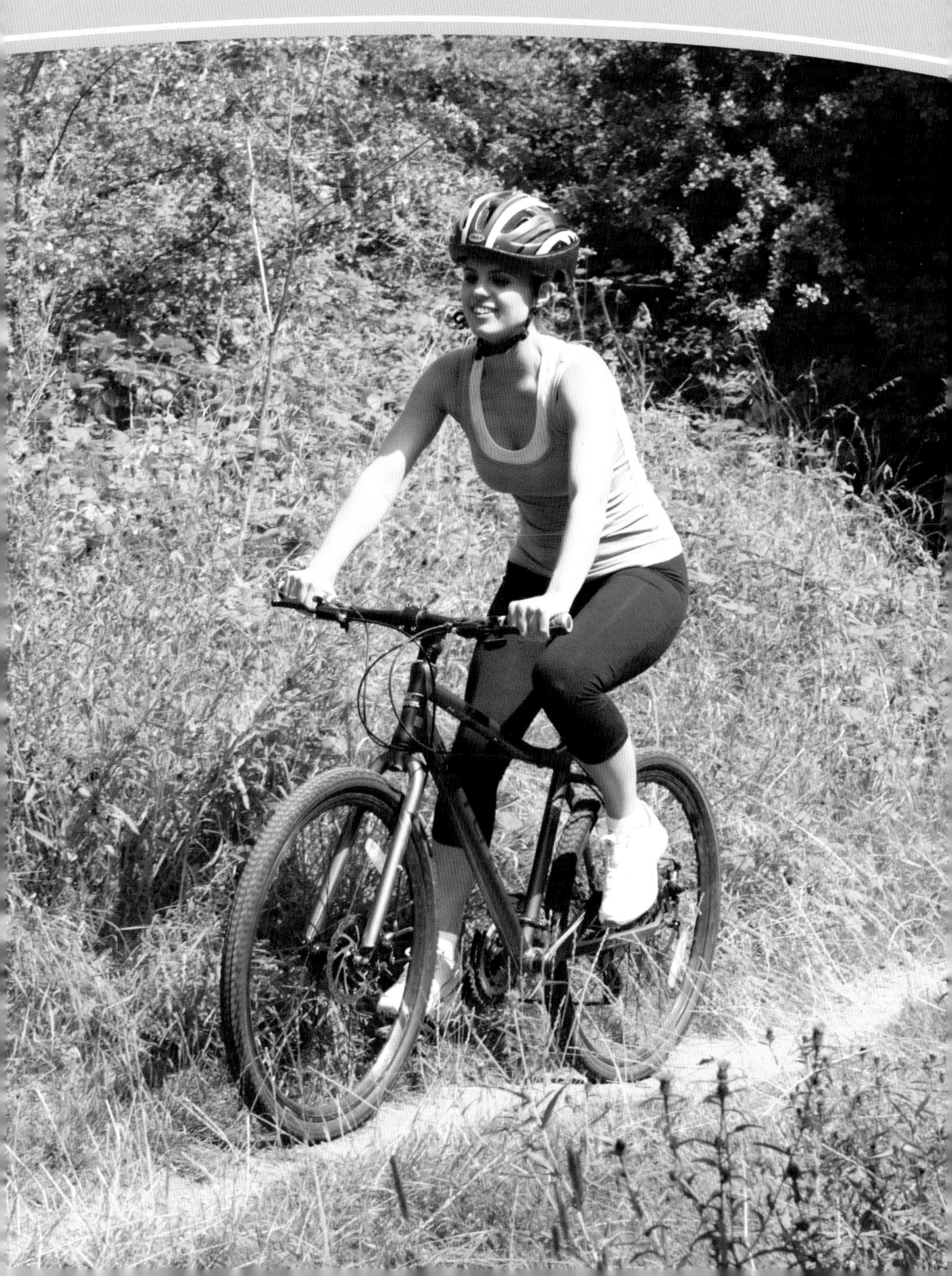

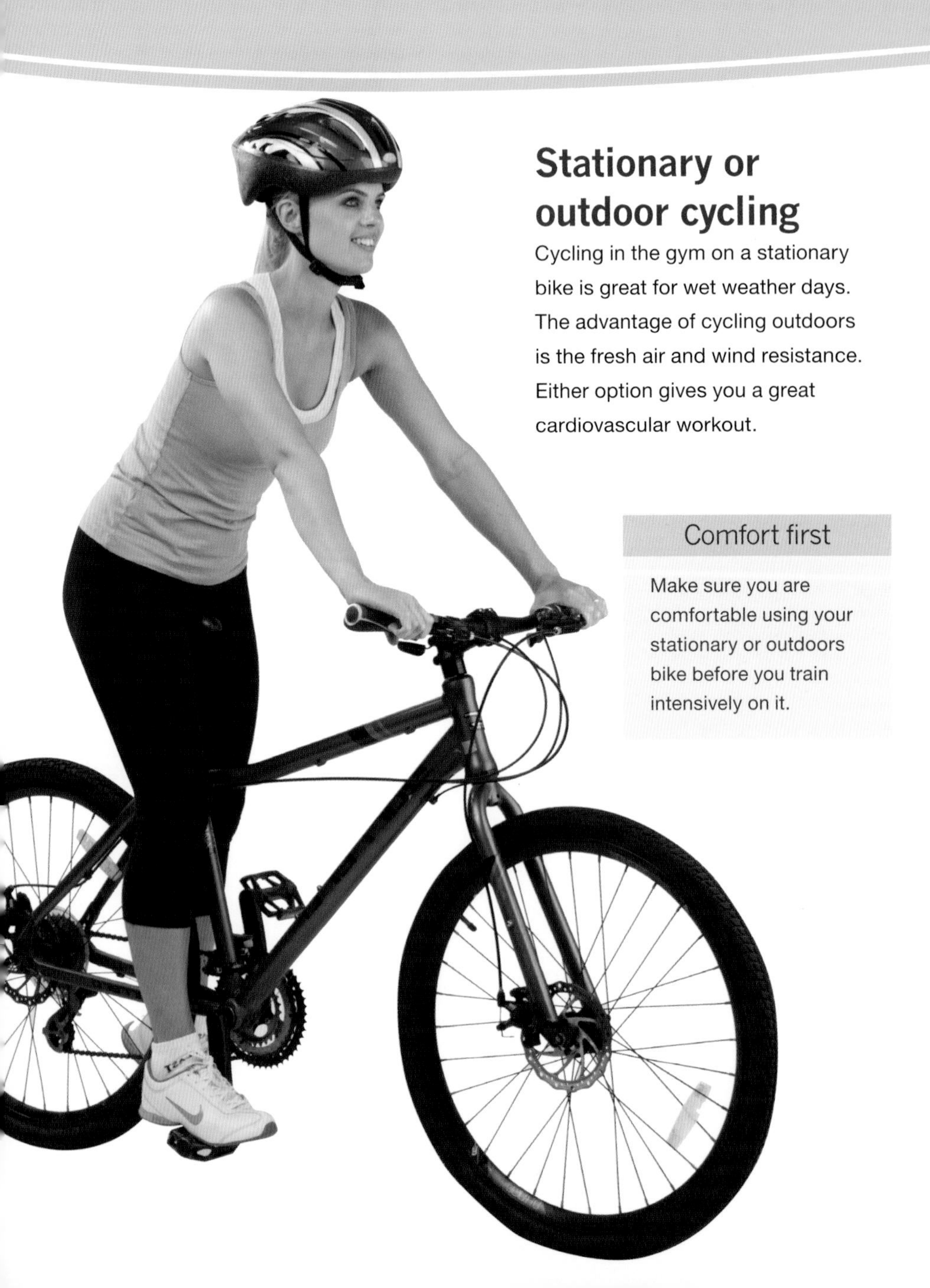

Stationary or outdoor cycling

Cycling in the gym on a stationary bike is great for wet weather days. The advantage of cycling outdoors is the fresh air and wind resistance. Either option gives you a great cardiovascular workout.

Comfort first

Make sure you are comfortable using your stationary or outdoors bike before you train intensively on it.

The bike

Adjust the bike so it suits you, not the much taller or shorter person who was on it before you in the gym! Move the seat so it is at the correct height, as this will keep your posture strong.

Ideally, you will use a stationary bike that has settings to vary the resistance. As well as setting the resistance level of the bike, vary the cadence (the number of revolutions per minute, rpm) that you are cycling. As a guide, 80 rpm is a moderate level and 100 rpm intense.

Workout

A: Total time 14 minutes

2 minute warm-up

30 seconds at 90 rpm

2 minutes recovery

Repeat 4 times

2 minute cool-down and stretch out

B: Total time 14 minutes

2 minute warm-up

30 seconds at 100 rpm

2 minutes recovery

Repeat 4 times

2 minute cool-down and stretch out

C: Total time 14 minutes 40 seconds

2 minute warm-up

40 seconds at 100 rpm

2 minutes recovery

Repeat 4 times

2 minute cool-down and stretch out

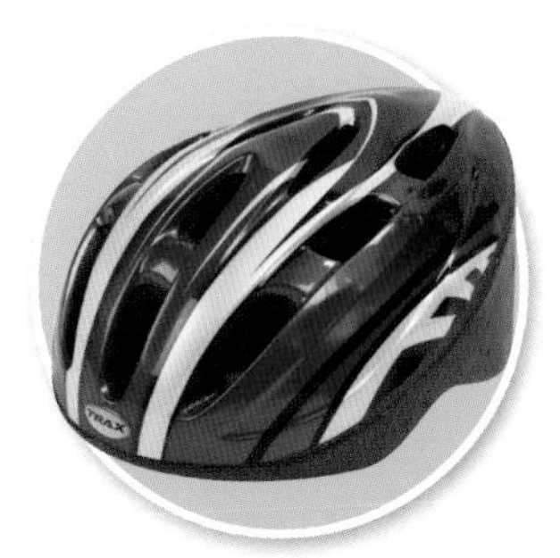

Uphill

For a seriously hard, intense workout, take any of the cycling routines but cycle uphill. Top tip – unless you are superhuman, don't start the intensive activity halfway up a hill! Start at the foot of the hill.

Standing and sitting

If you stand up to cycle, you apply force to the pedals using your whole body weight to drive them forward. Keep your back straight and shoulders down. You can't cycle standing for long periods, so save it for the hills.

Gear up

Use your gears to increase or decrease the intensity. Switching to a higher gear increases resistance and makes you work harder. Push your workout to the maximum (this is advanced) by moving to a high gear going uphill.

Cycling (before an intense workout) uses up an amazing 600 calories per hour. It works the legs and is kinder on the knees than running. However, there are important stretches that a cyclist should do. Work your shoulders, quadriceps and hamstrings.

A yoga pose called Downward Dog is an excellent stretch for the back muscles and hamstrings in one go. If you prefer, you can use a more traditional stretch for your calves and hamstrings – as shown opposite.

Can't beat beetroot!

You may have heard rumours of an amazing tonic that helps the Tour de France competitors pedal the course – it's beetroot! Beet juice is full of nitrates, which widen blood vessels to allow more blood flow and reduces the amount of oxygen needed by muscles during activity.

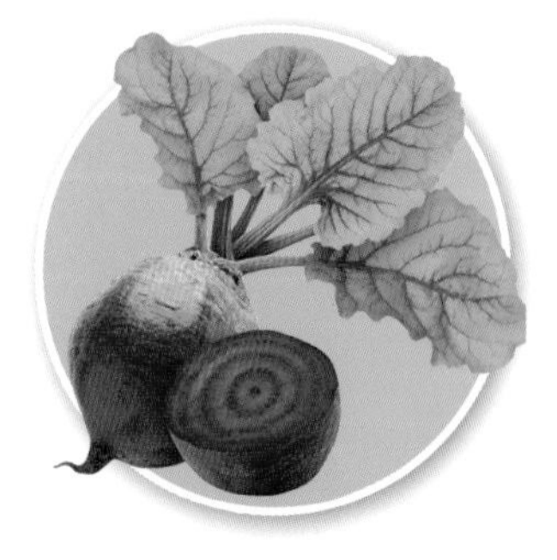

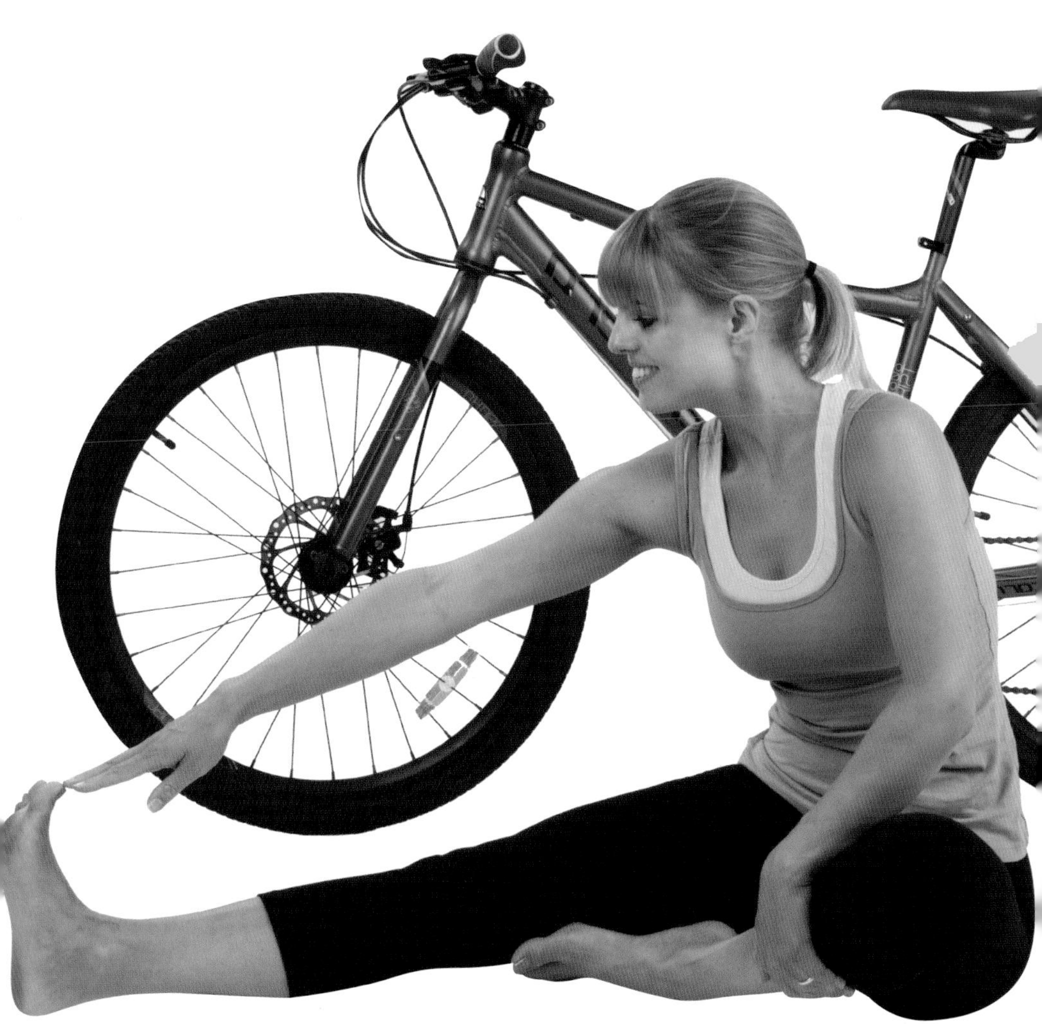

pre-cycle stretch

Swimming

Swimming is an excellent workout that uses all of the muscles in your body, and it's low impact, so kind on the joints. As water is denser (heavier) than air, there is ready-made resistance in the pool with your every move.

You'll need a pair of goggles. Take a water bottle with you and keep it at one end of the pool – you will need it!

Warm up

Do your warm-up by the side of the pool and in the pool.

Stretch your arms and shoulders

- Bring one arm across your chest
- Hold it gently at the elbow with your other hand, pulling it towards your chest
- Repeat on the other side

Stretch your upper arm

- Lift one bent elbow into the air, by your head
- Cross your other arm over your head and at the elbow gently pull your arm. Swap arms and repeat

Neck rolls

- Gently roll your head around clockwise and anticlockwise

Warm up legs

- Tread water for 60 seconds
- Gently swim a few laps

Your warm-up time will depend on the speed at which you swim gently or moderately. As a general rule, a four minute warm-up swim will get your muscles ready for the workout.

For your recovery, swim at a gentle or moderate pace.

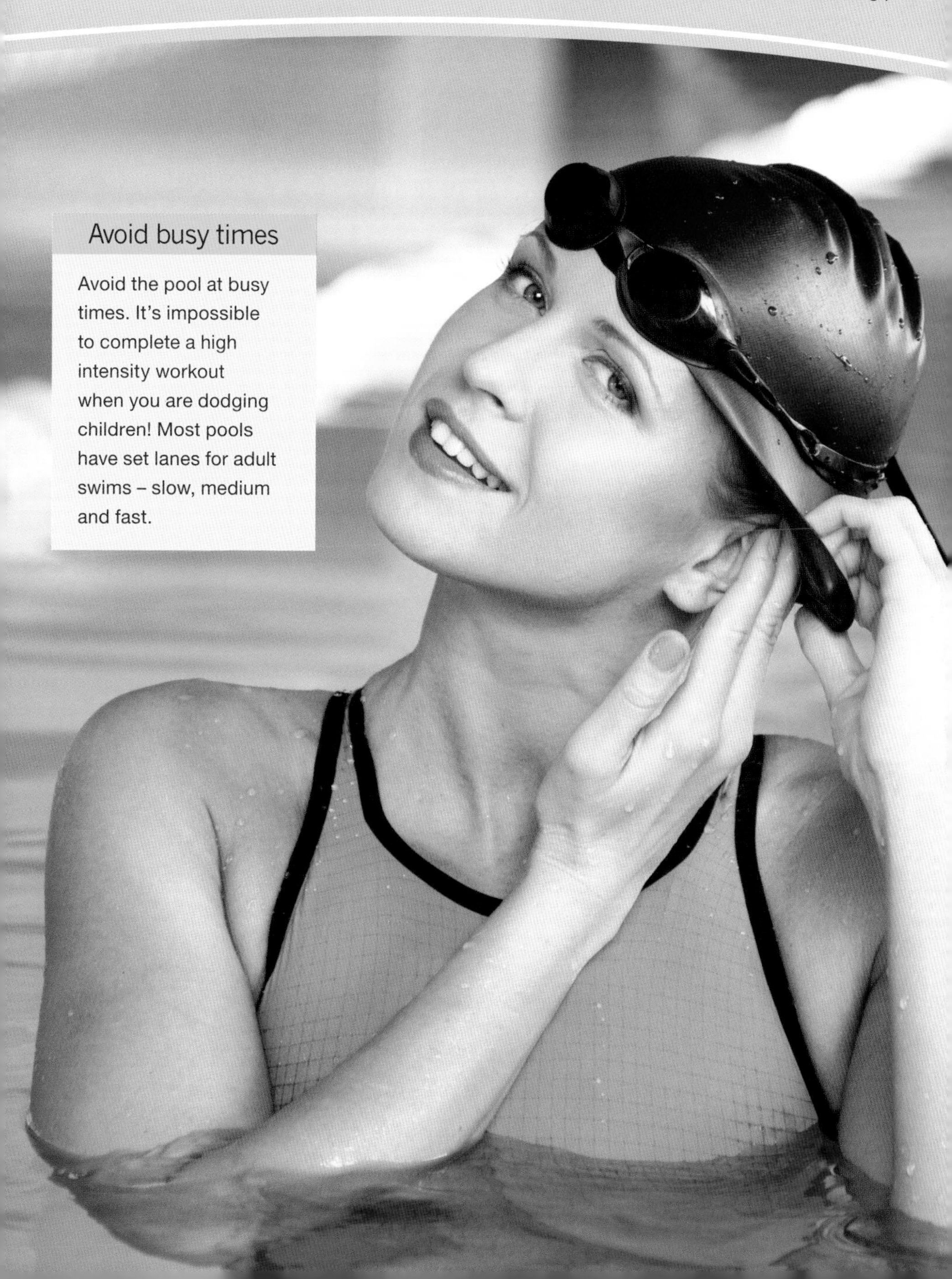

Avoid busy times

Avoid the pool at busy times. It's impossible to complete a high intensity workout when you are dodging children! Most pools have set lanes for adult swims – slow, medium and fast.

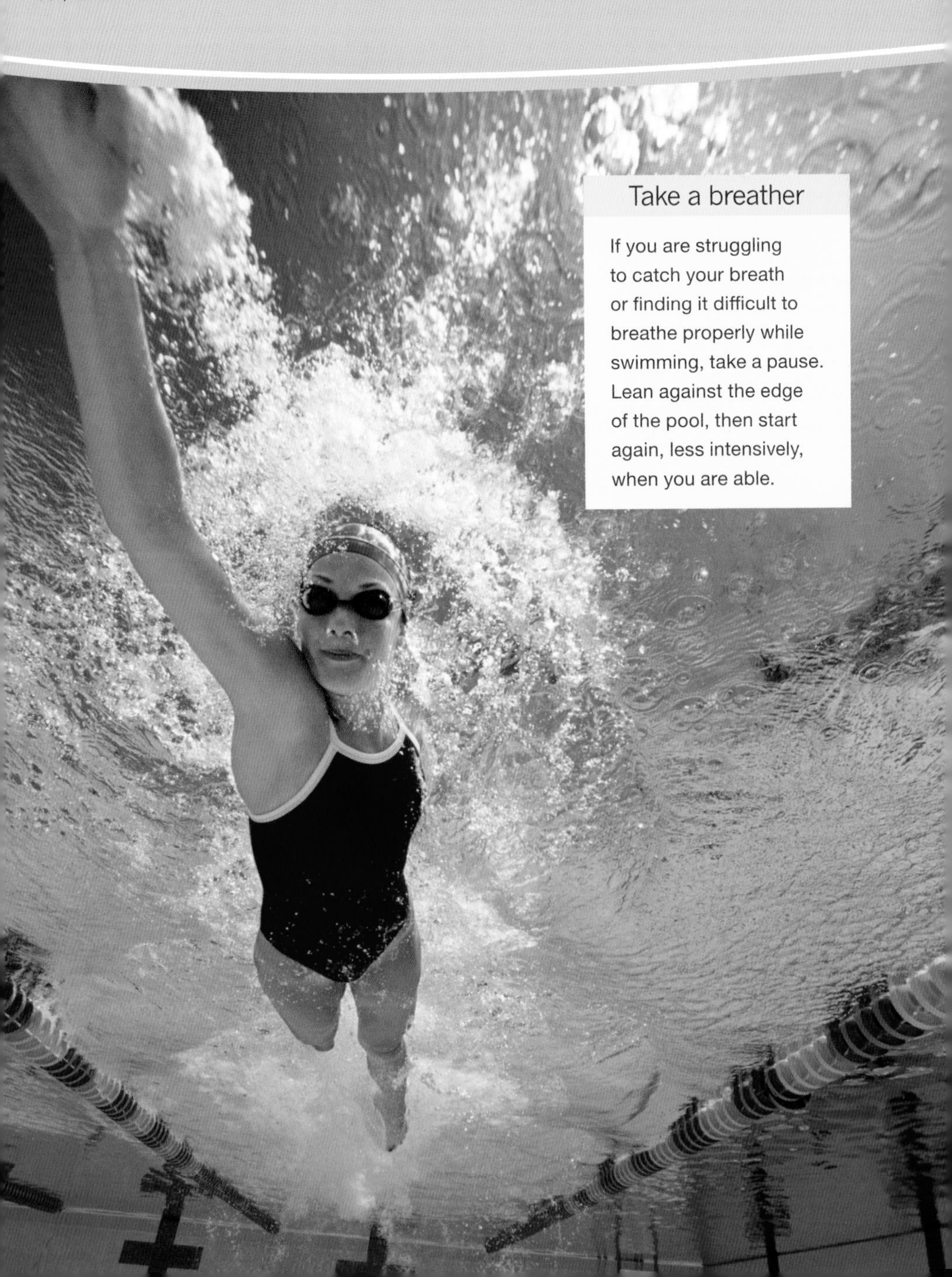

Take a breather

If you are struggling to catch your breath or finding it difficult to breathe properly while swimming, take a pause. Lean against the edge of the pool, then start again, less intensively, when you are able.

Workout

It's not as easy in a pool to measure time, so it may be easier to work out roughly the distance that you need to cover in high intensity.

A: Total time 9 minutes 20 seconds

4 minute warm-up

20 seconds swim (high intensity)

80 seconds recovery

Repeat 2 times

2 minute cool-down and stretch

To begin, aim to work at 75 per cent of your maximum. Build up gradually.

B: Total time 10 minutes 30 seconds

4 minute warm-up

30 seconds swim

60 seconds recovery

Repeat 3 times

2 minute cool-down and stretch

C: Total time 11 minutes

4 minute warm-up

40 seconds swim

60 seconds recovery

Repeat 3 times

2 minute cool-down and stretch

D: Total time 16 minutes

4 minute warm-up

60 seconds swim

2 minutes recovery

Start with 4 reps; gradually aim to build up to 10

2 minute cool-down and stretch

Repeat the above, and aim to work at 80 per cent of your maximum intensity. Don't forget your recovery periods – they are crucial.

Strokes

When you are working fast in the pool, decide on your strokes before you start. Make your workout more interesting by mixing up your strokes (but not during the middle of a burst).

Front crawl

This is the stroke that works your upper body and is used most often in competitive swimming because it is the most efficient. Hold your abdominals tight. Use your shoulder to power your arm movements and think about extending your arms rather than crashing them down.

Breaststroke

This is great for your hips and inner thigh muscles. It also works your chest muscles. Before you start with this stroke, make sure you are comfortable with your head in the water – goggles make all the difference here. Swimming with your head out of the water and at an angle to the rest of the body will cause neck problems.

Backstroke

This gives you a welcome chance to have your face and eyes out of the water and breathe normally! More importantly, backstroke works your back and shoulder muscles. Relax your neck and head and aim to look just above your feet, not at the ceiling. Make sure you have a clear path in the pool, otherwise you will crash into another swimmer.

Butterfly

This stroke, shown on the opposite page, is one of the hardest strokes and works on upper body strength and stretches the body. Doing this at high intensity is advanced.

How hard is hard?

If you feel you could easily swim for another 20 seconds at the end of your high intensity swim, then you need to increase your effort. Try swimming the same amount of time but putting in extra push. As a target, aim to cover more distance in the same time, or cover the same distance in less time.

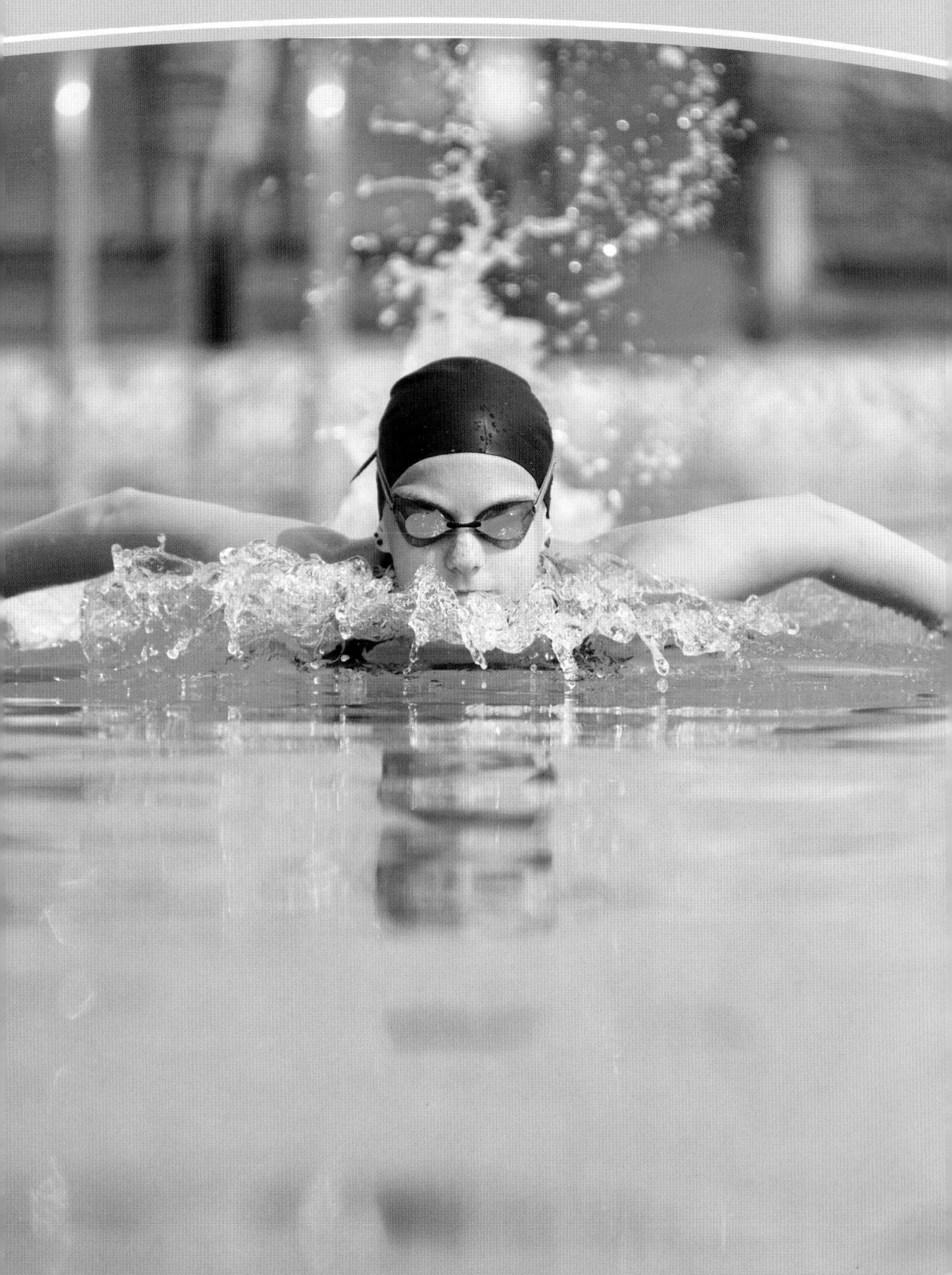

Social swimming

Make your workout more fun and challenging by working out in the pool with a friend. One swims fast, while the other swims gently or treads water, counting and generally encouraging the high intensity swimmer. Then swap and repeat the workout.

Swimming lessons

As with any exercise, the better your technique, the more effective your workout. Swimming doesn't come as naturally to most of us as cycling or running, so it may be worth investing in a couple of swimming lessons.

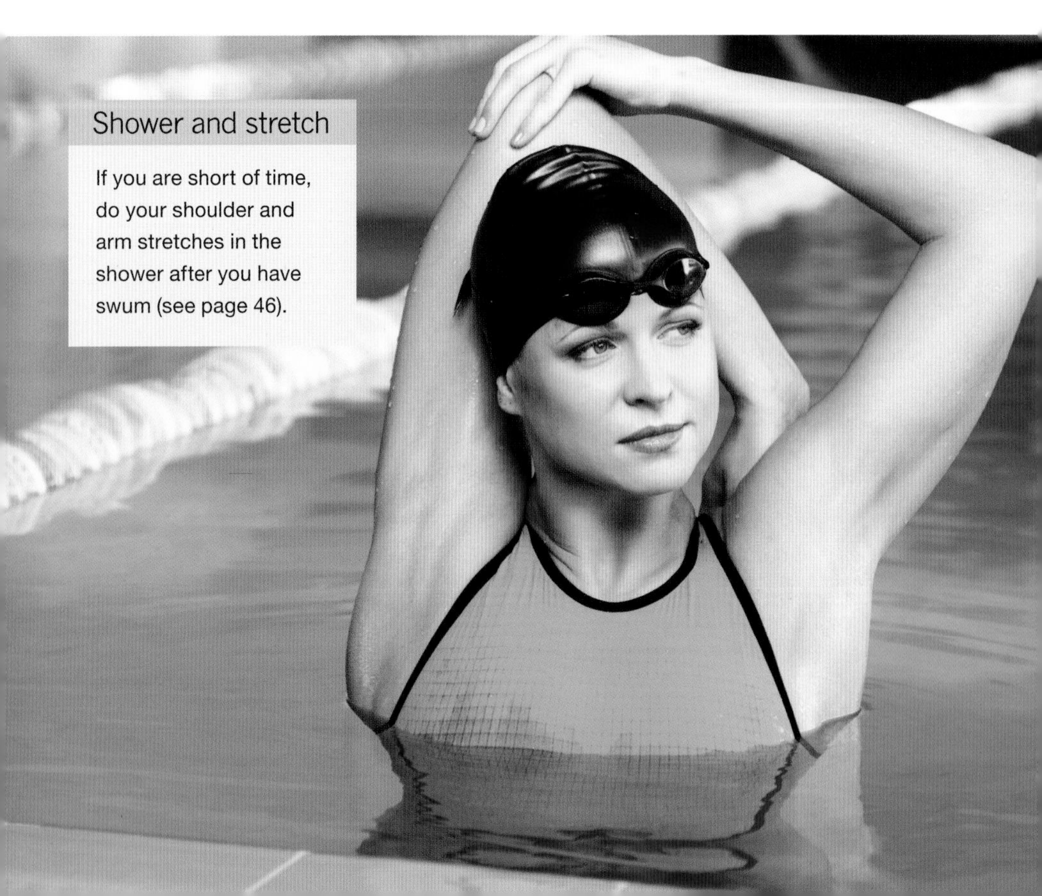

Shower and stretch

If you are short of time, do your shoulder and arm stretches in the shower after you have swum (see page 46).

Non-swimmer workouts

There are ways of working out in water at high intensity even if you are not a swimmer. Work in the shallow end. With all of the following, work hard to reap the rewards of fast fitness, but keep the movements strong and controlled. Start off with 30 seconds, exercise and 60 seconds' rest. Repeat at least four times and then add duration and repetition to the set.

Tread

- Tread water while swinging your arms

- Then tread water with your arms across your chest

Bicycle

- Lean back against the side of the pool with your arms stretched out to your sides. Hold the edge of the pool

- Pedal your legs as fast as you can

Push

- In the same starting position as bicycle, instead of pedalling in a circular motion, push both your legs out with maximum force and bring them back into your chest

Pull up

- Hold on to the side of the pool

- Lower your body into the water, with your arms extended. Use your arms to pull you up and lower down again

Hip out

- Facing the side of the pool, hold on with both hands

- Extend one leg out to the side with your foot flexed and turned at 90 degrees to the pool side. Repeat this at speed but with control, 20 times per leg

Circuits

Circuits can be done anywhere: at home, in the gym, in the park. You don't need any special equipment and can improvise with what is at hand. The point about circuits is to include a range of exercises that will give your body a good workout, top to toe. Working within fast fitness, focus on a few exercises in one session that work different parts of your body. Vary the exercises for your next session. Warm up with some gentle jogging for two minutes and do some stretches that are appropriate for the area you will be working. The pattern of fast circuits will be different from running, cycling and swimming because you are including more than one activity. Aim for a one minute rest between each.

Star jumps

- Stand straight with your arms by your sides

- Bend your knees

- As you jump up, open your arms and legs wide into a star shape, while you are in the air

- Land with your legs apart and knees slightly bent

Star jump workout

20 seconds star jumps

60 seconds recovery

Repeat 4 times

For a more advanced jump, vary the landing:

- Land with your knees closer together and low enough so you can touch the floor with your hands. From this position, spring back up. Exercise for 30 seconds and rest for 60 seconds. Repeat 4 times

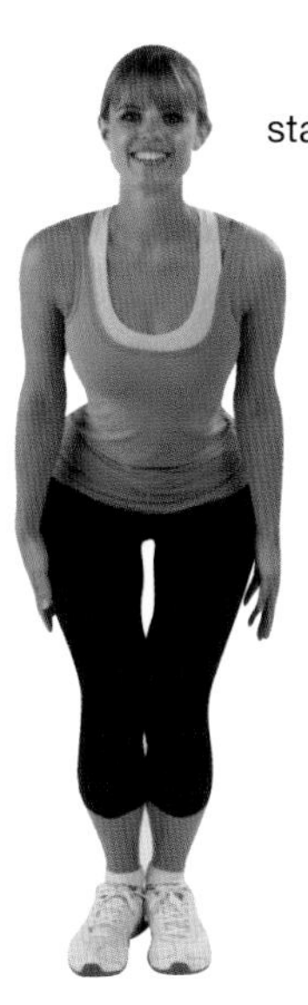

star jump

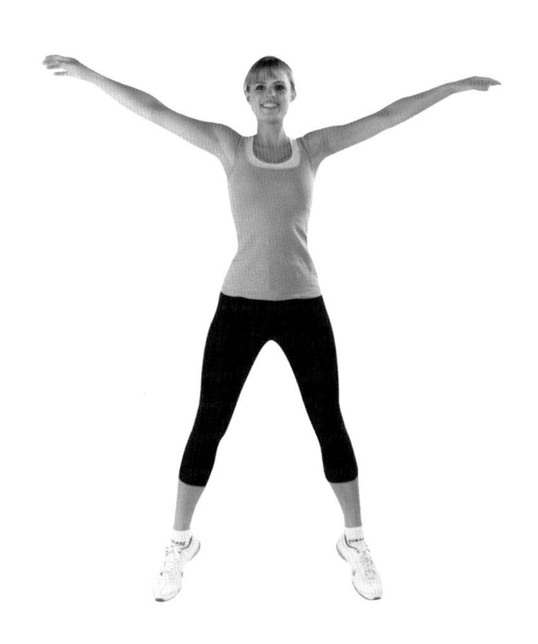

advanced
star jump

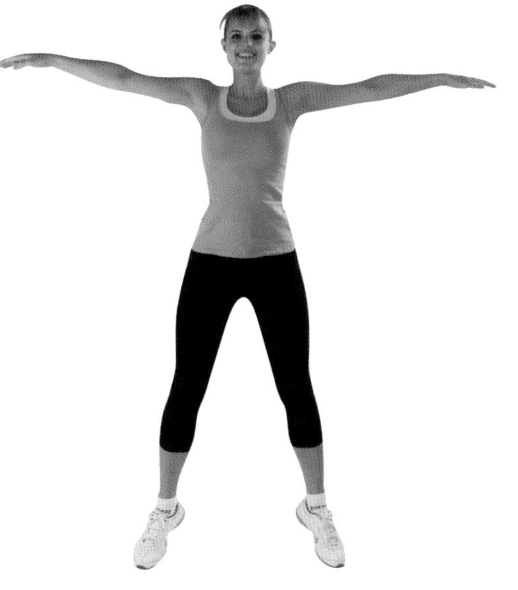

Squat!

- Stand with your feet shoulder-width apart, feet facing forwards
- Stretch your hands out in front
- Bend your knees to lower your body, as though you are going to sit down
- Keep your back straight, abdominals tight
- Aim to have your thighs parallel to the floor but don't let your knees come over your toes
- With control, return to the starting position

Squat workout

30 seconds of squats

60 seconds recovery

Repeat 4 times

Kick and squat

Add a kick to your squats

- Lower into a squat
- As you push up, kick out forwards with one leg. Keep it controlled
- Lower into a squat and come up to kick with the other leg

Kick and squat Workout

30 seconds kick and squats

60 seconds recovery

Repeat 4 times

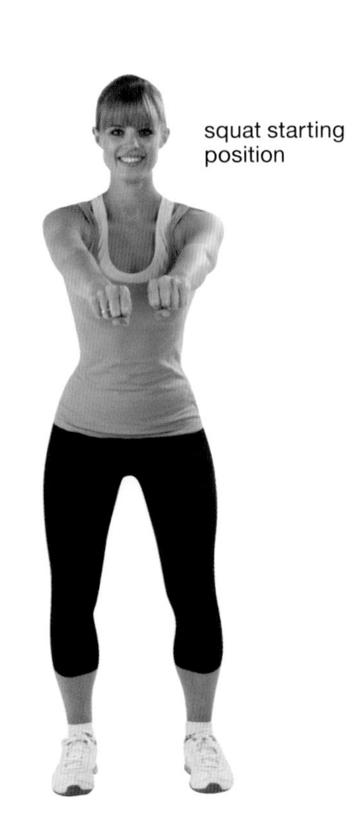

squat starting position

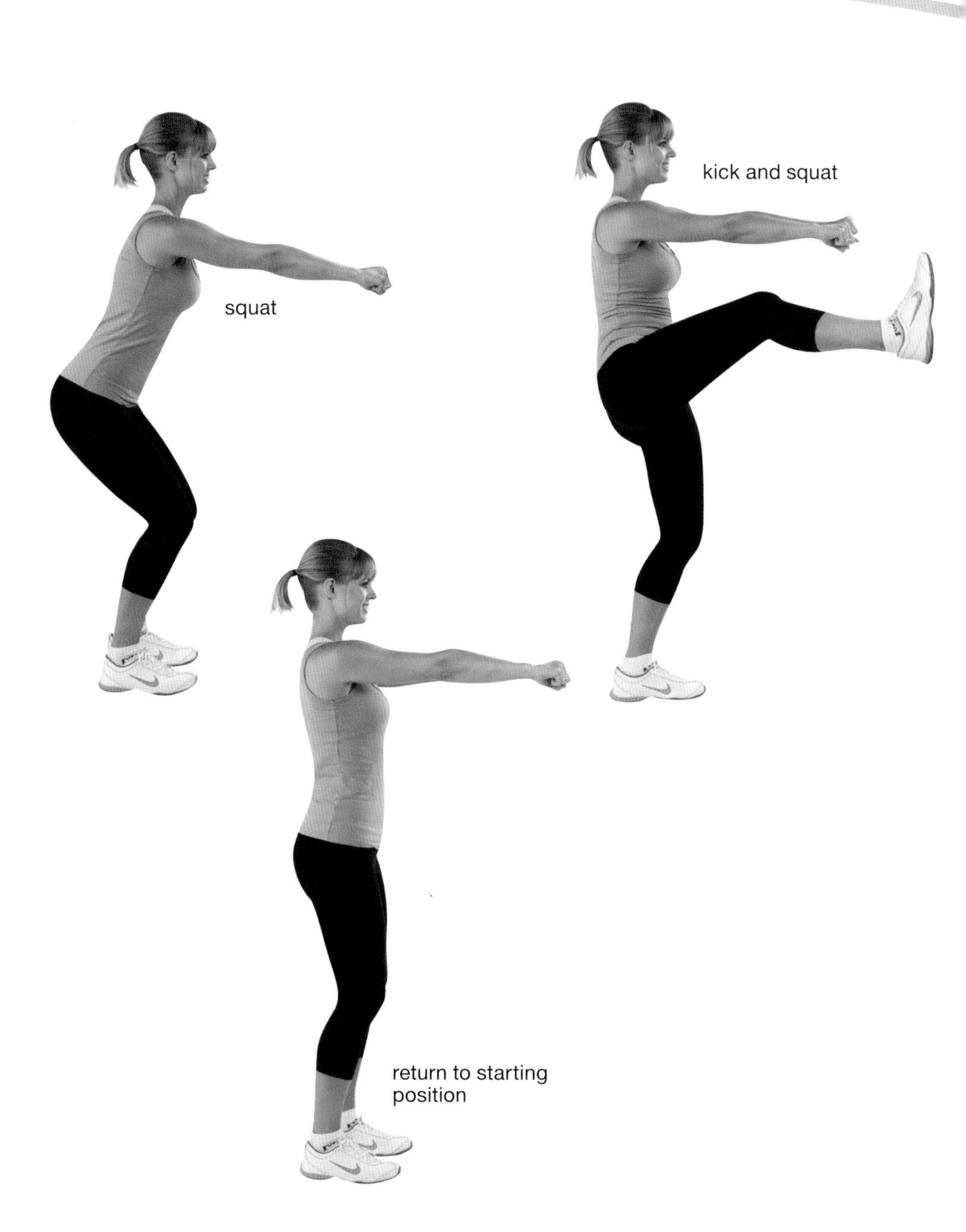
squat
kick and squat
return to starting position

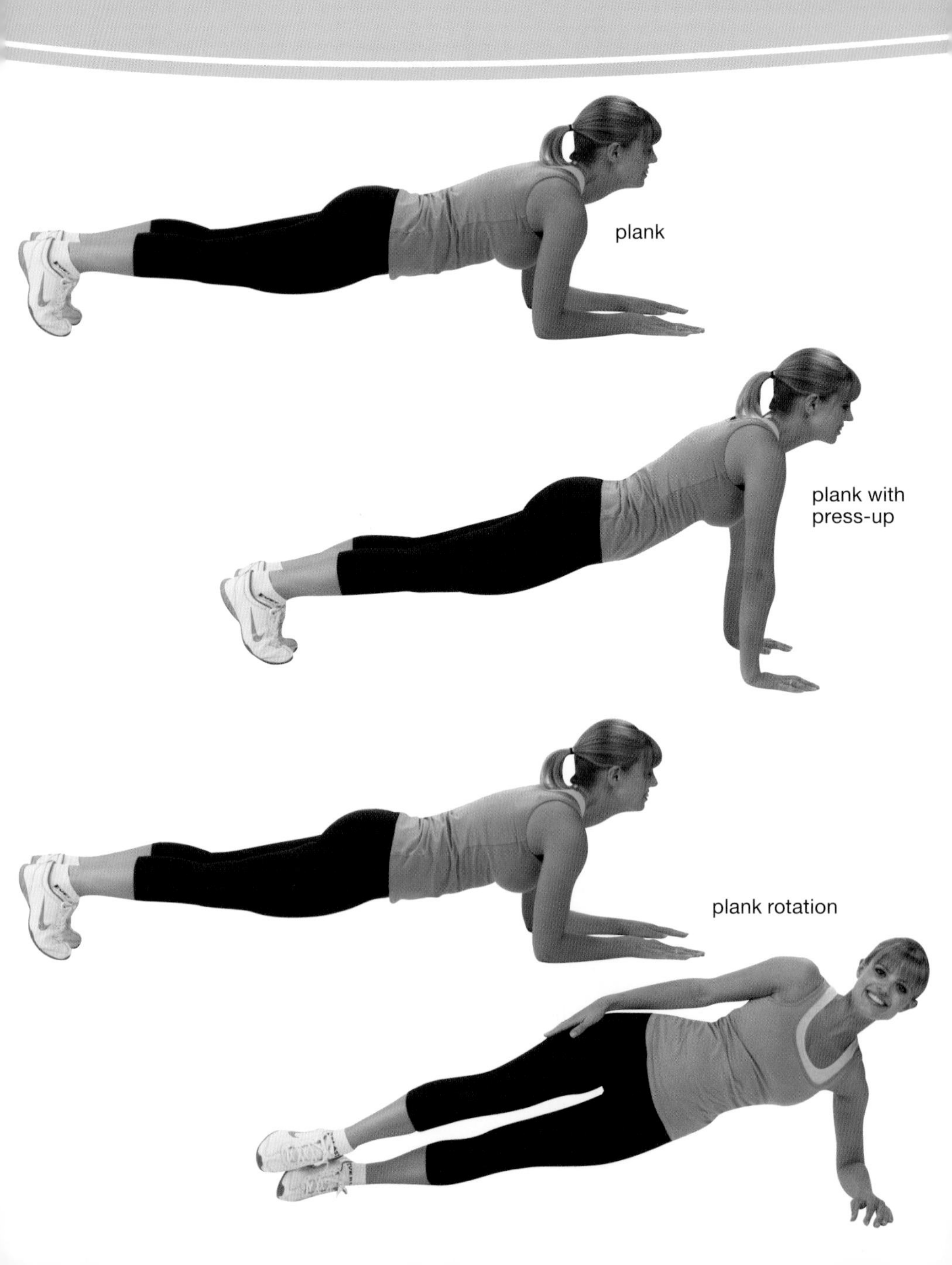
plank
plank with
press-up
plank rotation

Plank

Work your upper body, abdominals, lower back and buttocks with the super-effective plank. Start in a press-up position. Bend your elbows with your weight on your forearms (your arms are to your sides). Hold your abdominals tight and keep your body in a straight line from your shoulders to ankles.

Variations in plank

- Perform a press-up (or several) while in plank
- Rotate from plank on to one side, keeping your weight on one forearm. Keep your body in a straight line. Rotate from here to the other side

Lunge

Lunges work your abdominals, hips and legs. See opposite for the correct lunging position.

- Stand with your back straight and your feet shoulder-width apart
- Bring one leg forward, bending both knees at right angles. Land with the heel of your front foot first and then bring the ball of your foot down
- Bring the front leg back and repeat on the other side

Jump lunges

These lunges will really get your heart pumping.

- From a lunge position, push up with your front leg
- Mid-air, switch legs and land with the opposite leg forward

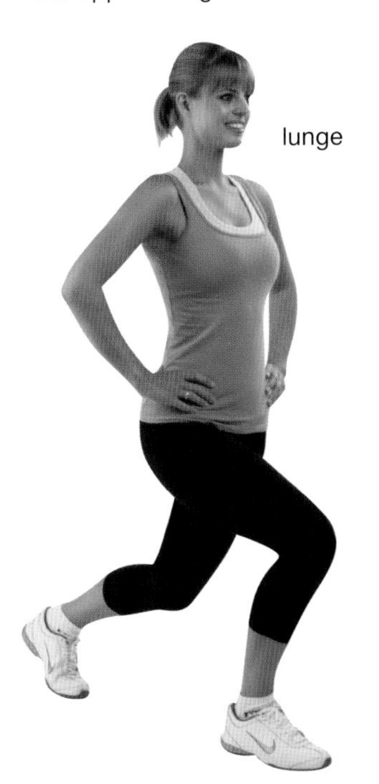

lunge

Tricep dip

Your triceps are the muscles at the back of your upper arm.

- Sit on the floor with your back to a bench or chair – make sure it is not going to tip over or move
- Put your hands shoulder-width apart on the bench or chair with your fingers pointing towards you
- Lift your buttocks off the ground and straighten your legs (heels remain on the ground)
- Bend your elbows behind you so that you lower your backside to the ground
- Push back up until your elbows are straight

Stairway to fitness

Fast fitness on the stairs: sounds too easy to be true, but once you've run up those stairs several times you will know it's high intensity and that it isn't easy! Just make sure the stairs are not being used by other people as you bound up and down – and be careful.

- Run up the stairs safely as many times as you can within two minutes. Walk down. (Obviously, you need to be sensible – if it is a very high or low set of stairs, adapt your timings)

Skip

Skipping is a great cardiovascular workout. To check your rope is the correct length, stand on the middle of the rope and pull the handles upwards until the rope is taut. The handles should be chest height. Wear trainers when you skip to provide a cushioned and supported landing. Keep your head up and try to land lightly on your toes. Keep your elbows in at the side. Getting the technique right takes practice.

- Skip for 30 seconds
- Rest (jog lightly on the spot) for 60 seconds

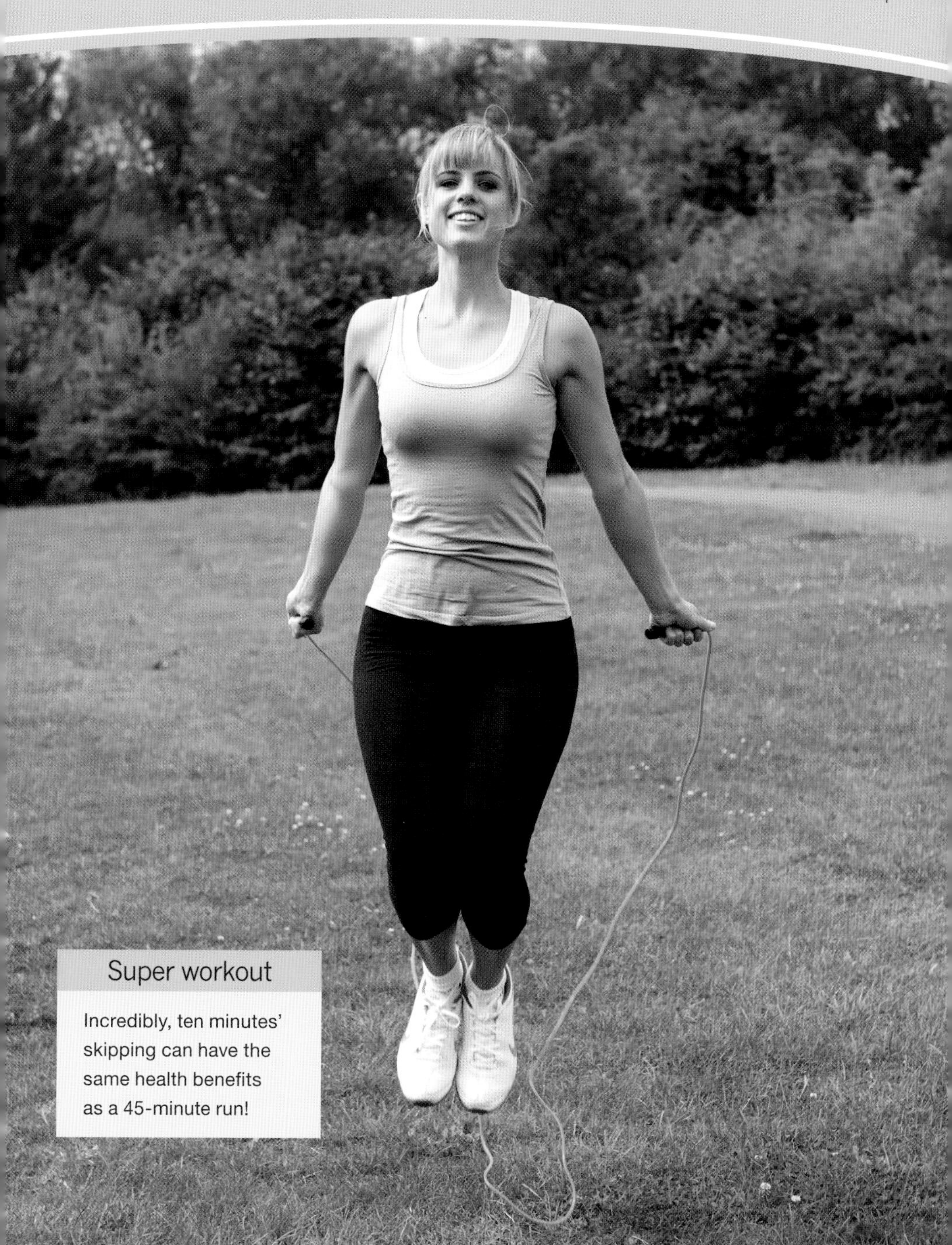

Super workout

Incredibly, ten minutes' skipping can have the same health benefits as a 45-minute run!

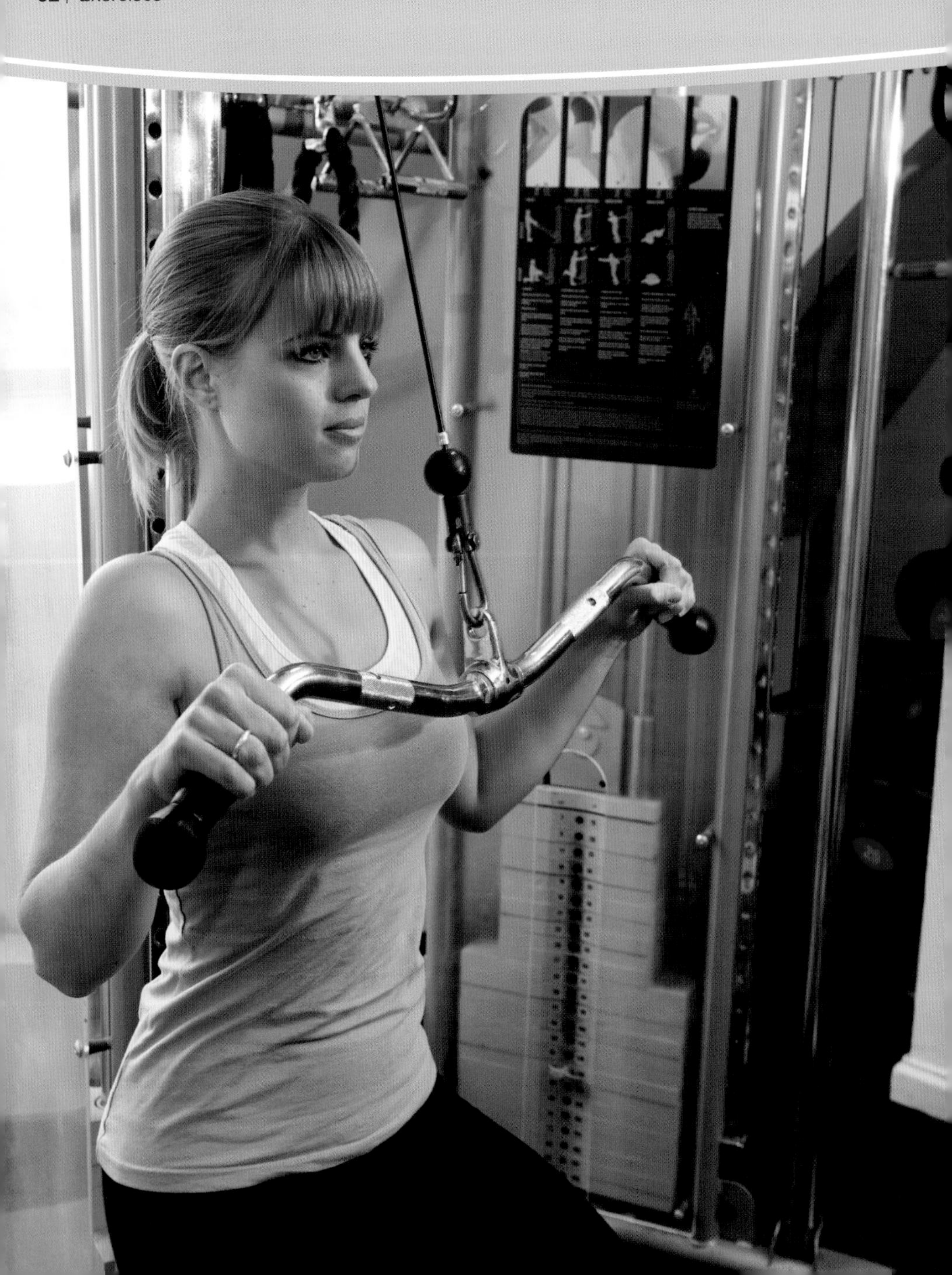

Weighty Work

A lot of women associate weights with building bulky muscles. However, unless you continue to lift heavy weights once you have reached your desired shape, you won't bulk up.

You can use weight-training exercises at home or in the gym as part of your circuit session. If you are working in a gym, you will need an induction by the gym staff to show you how to use the equipment safely. If you haven't got the time to go to a gym, you can perform these exercises at home, in the office or in the park. Get lifting!

At home, you can use bags of sugar or tins of food as your lifts for upper body work but, you may prefer to invest in some weights. Dumbbells are hand-held weights that increase the intensity of exercises such as lunges, squats and bicep curls. A barbell is a long bar with circular weights at each end. When you use weights you greatly increase the intensity of the strength-training exercises in your workout.

Using weights mainly works on your strength, but if you perform the exercises in this chapter at high intensity and add in some cardiovascular exercises, such as skipping or stair running, you will also be working on your cardiovascular fitness.

Performed to the full, these weight exercises will make your limbs tremble with the effort. This shouldn't be painful though, and if it is, stop. In addition, it is not a good idea to exercise hard with an injury as it will only worsen it and prolong recovery.

There are a few important points to keep in mind. When you give the weight workouts a try, always warm up first with some gentle jogging and stretching. To keep things interesting, maintain your motivation and challenge yourself, vary the duration and number of repetitions. Lastly, don't miss out the recovery and rest times.

Single arm rows

- Position yourself on all fours
- With one hand, pick up your weight
- Lift the weight up towards the side of the chest, bending the elbow and bringing your hand to your chest
- Keep your back flat and straight, and lower the weight to the floor
- Repeat on the other arm

Shoulder press

- Sit on a chair or stand with your feet hip-width apart. Keep your abdominals tight
- Hold a weight in either hand, by your shoulders, elbows bent
- Push up directly overhead, with your arms straightened. With a controlled movement, lower them to the starting position
- Repeat 10 times

Shoulder raises

- Stand tall with your feet shoulder-width apart
- Hold the weights to the side of your shoulders, at shoulder height
- Push upwards, raising the weights into the air
- Controlling the movement, lower the weights to shoulder level
- Repeat 10 times

For each of these exercises, begin with 10 reps on each side followed by 30 seconds recovery. Repeat the routine three times.

To challenge yourself further, aim for 40 seconds lifting followed by 60 seconds recovery, repeated three times.

Muscle burns fat

Gram for gram, muscle burns more calories than fat. If you increase your muscle mass, you greatly increase your fat-burning capacity, meaning that even when you are not exercising you are burning fat.

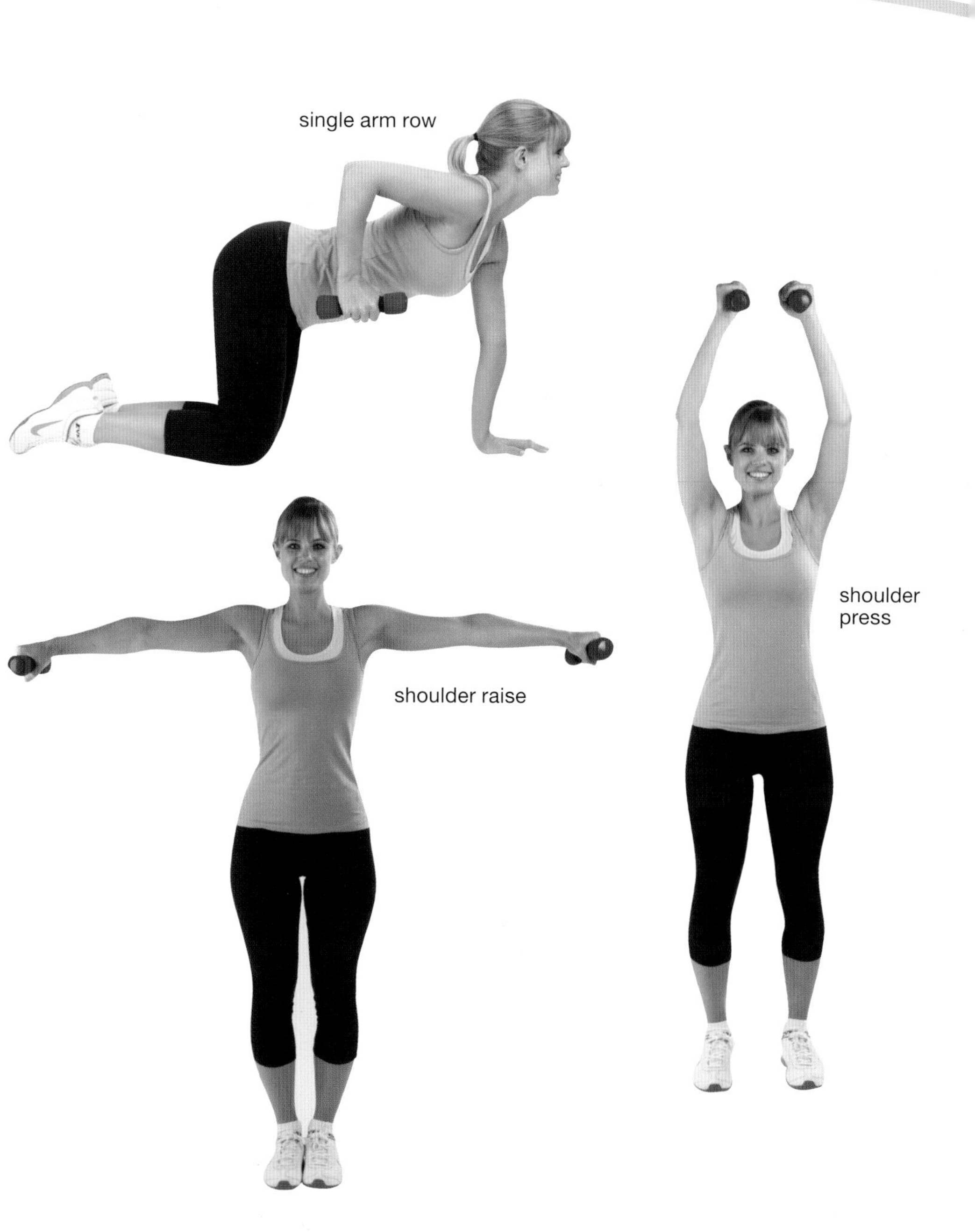
single arm row
shoulder press
shoulder raise

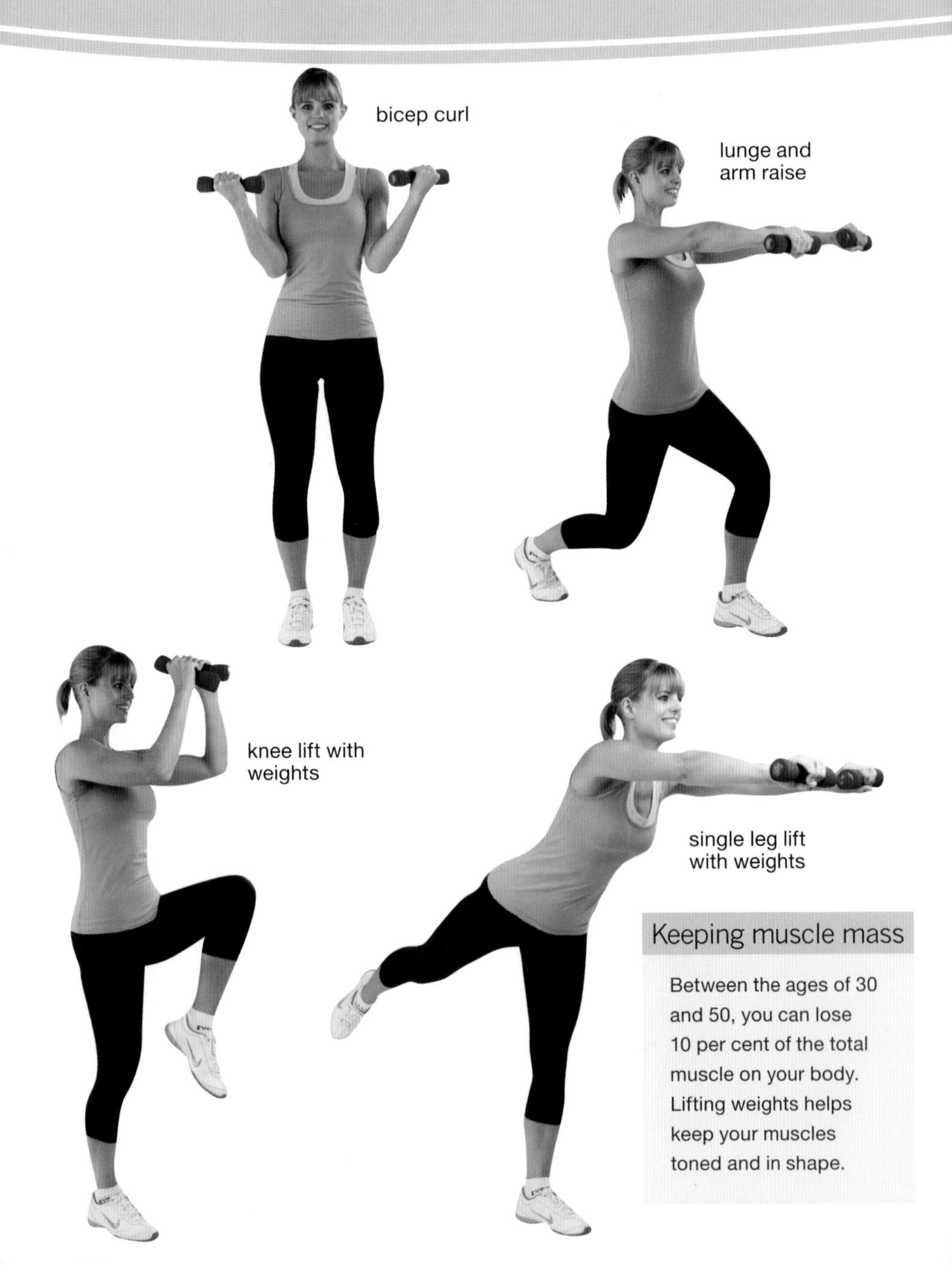

Keeping muscle mass

Between the ages of 30 and 50, you can lose 10 per cent of the total muscle on your body. Lifting weights helps keep your muscles toned and in shape.

Bicep curl

Your bicep is the muscle at the front of your upper arm.

- Hold the weights by your thighs. Bend your elbow, lift them to shoulder height and control the descent
- Add this to walking up the stairs very briskly, but be careful not to trip. It can be quite difficult to get the co-ordination correct

Lunge and arm raise

This is a hard exercise that will work both your upper and lower body.

- Stand tall with a weight in each hand
- Lunge forwards, keeping your arms straight
- Lift the arms up to your shoulders, keeping the elbow straight. Repeat for 10 reps and step back to your starting position
- Repeat on the other side

Knee lift with weights

- Hold your weights and extend your arms to shoulder height. Bend your elbows at 90 degrees
- As you lift each knee, bring your arms together in front of your chest
- Repeat 20 times

Single leg lift with weights

This works your hamstrings, buttocks and abdominals.

- Hold a weight in each hand and stand tall. Make sure your abdominals are tight
- Lean forward, keeping your back straight and extend your right leg. Control your arms as they extend in front of you – your arms and right leg are extended in a straight line
- Return to your starting position, squeezing your buttocks

Walking

Walking isn't usually up there when thinking about speedy weight loss and hard exercise. It's time to challenge that view. Put on some good walking shoes or running trainers and walk.

Stand tall

Posture is key to walking as an effective exercise. Aim for a straight vertical line from your ear to your ankle. Work your abdominal muscles and tuck your in bottom. Look forward. Swing your arms. Elbows should be bent at 90 degrees. Walking like this will work your arms and upper body, burn more calories and give you more momentum. Keep your shoulders relaxed. You don't need to swing your arms up to your face – swing them to chest level, and just beyond your hip.

Work those legs

- Hold your abdominals tight
- Pump your arms close to your body at a 90 degree angle
- Swing your arms to waist level
- Lead each step with your hip
- Place the heel of your front foot on the ground. Keep the front leg straight
- Put your foot in front of your body – it sounds obvious but it gives you the correct swing from the hip
- Use your toes to push off with your back foot, but try not to let your toes on the back foot leave the ground until the heel of the front foot is on the ground

Warm up with a regular walk of five minutes, swinging your arms. Practise the above before walking at speed. If you want to walk faster, increase your step rate rather than your stride length.

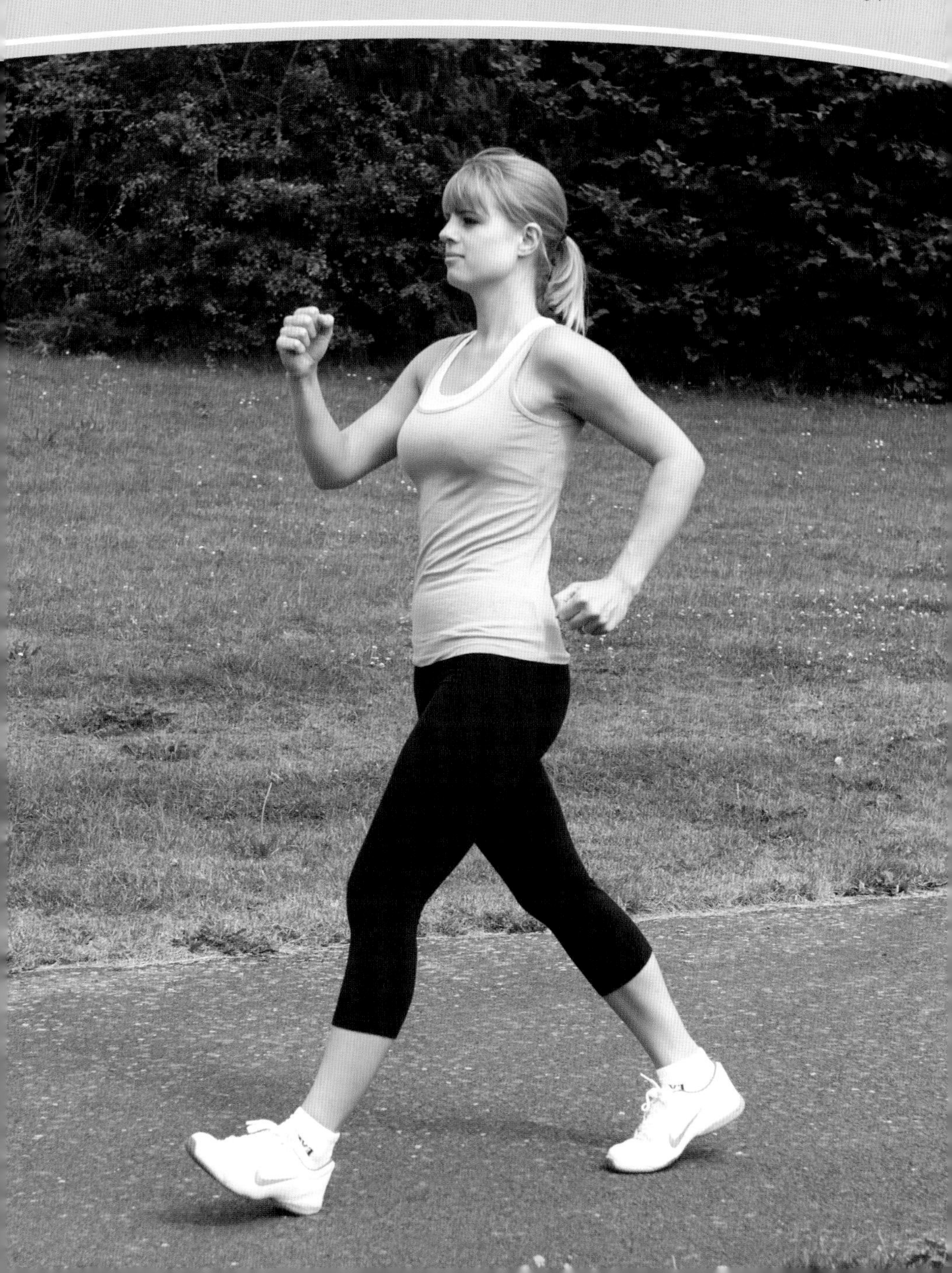

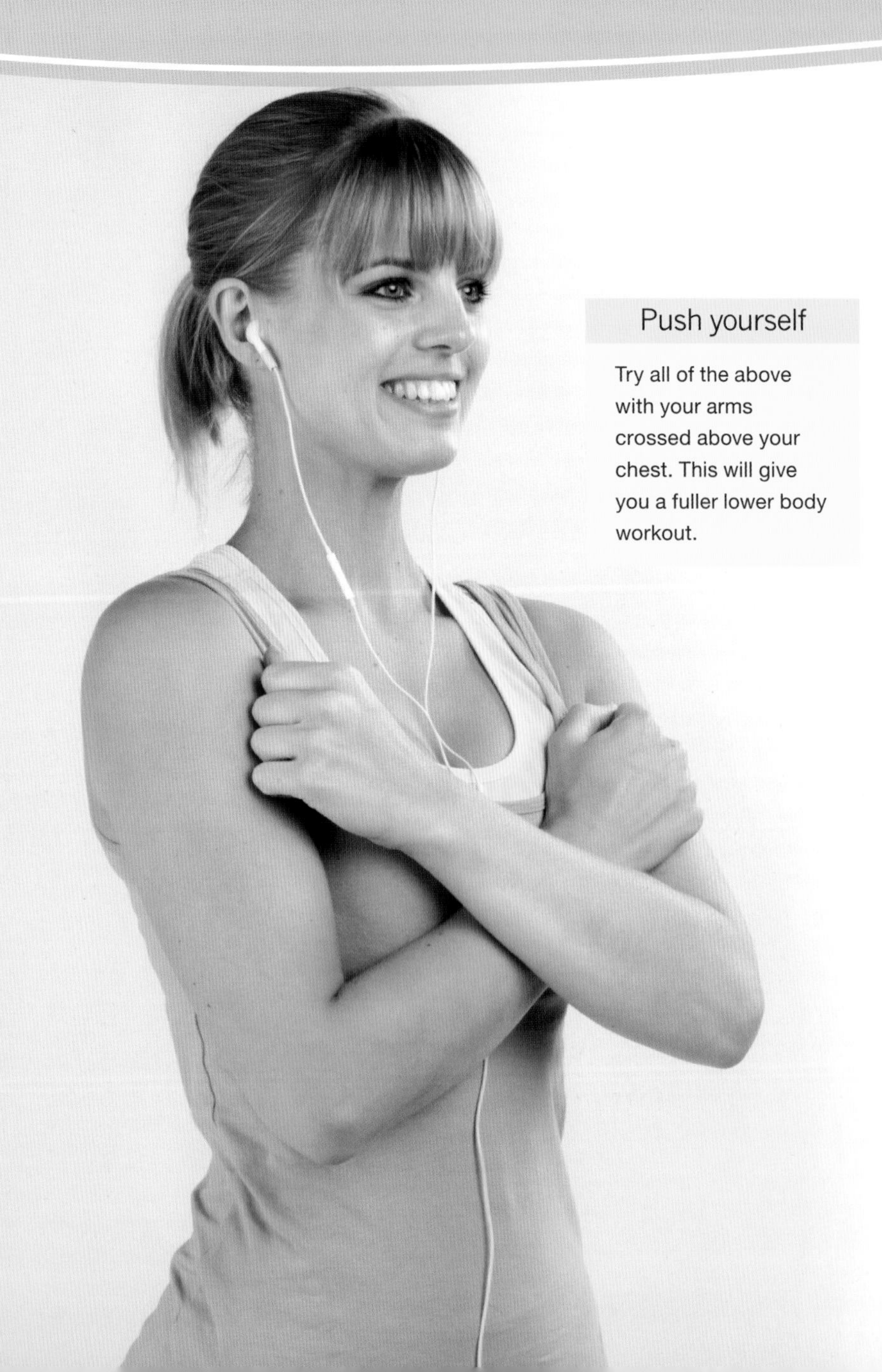

Push yourself

Try all of the above with your arms crossed above your chest. This will give you a fuller lower body workout.

Walk on

You've got the technique. Now it's time to get walking, fast. The duration of the high intensity workout is short but if you are walking with all your power, 30 seconds will be enough. Aim to walk with so much effort and vigour that you are unable to talk, should you want to! Warm up for between two and five minutes, take recovery periods and do a two-minute stretch at the end.

A: Total time 14 minutes 30 seconds

2 minute warm-up

30 seconds high intensity walk

3 minute recovery (gentle walking)

Repeat 3 times

2 minute cool-down and stretch out

B: Total time 16 minutes

2 minute warm-up

1 minute high intensity walk

2 minute recovery

Repeat 4 times

2 minute cool-down and stretch out

C: Total time 20 minutes

2 minute warm-up

2 minute high intensity walk

2 minute recovery

Repeat 4 times

2 minute cool-down and stretch out

Going uphill?

- Lean slightly into the hill but keep your weight over your hips
- Your natural stride length will be shorter, so in order to increase your speed, increase your step rate

Be cautious walking downhill – there is an increased risk of injuries.

Quick Fix

Try these quick fix exercises to work on particular problem areas, usually bums, thighs, tummies and arms.

The cardiovascular work of fast fitness will help reduce fat and improve tone, but the addition of strength training with exercises such as these will help significantly firm and shape up your bottom, abdominals, thighs and arms. You can do these for five or ten minutes.

Bums

These exercises work your gluteus maximus and minimus (often shortened to glutes). Try them for ten minutes for a shapely, toned bum.

Clench

- Lie on your back (ideally on a mat) with your knees bent and feet flat on the floor, shoulder-width apart
- Relax your neck. Squeeze your abs and buttocks to lift your hips
- Clench your buttocks as hard as you possibly can
- Gently lower the spine to the mat

Lift and extend

- In the same position as above (body in a straight line, hips up), lift and extend your left leg in line with your right thigh
- Squeeze your buttocks and lower your leg with control
- Repeat on the right leg
- Gently lower the spine to the mat

Donkey kick

- Start on all fours
- Extend your left leg. Lift and lower the extended leg for 10 reps
- Repeat 10 times, then repeat on the other side

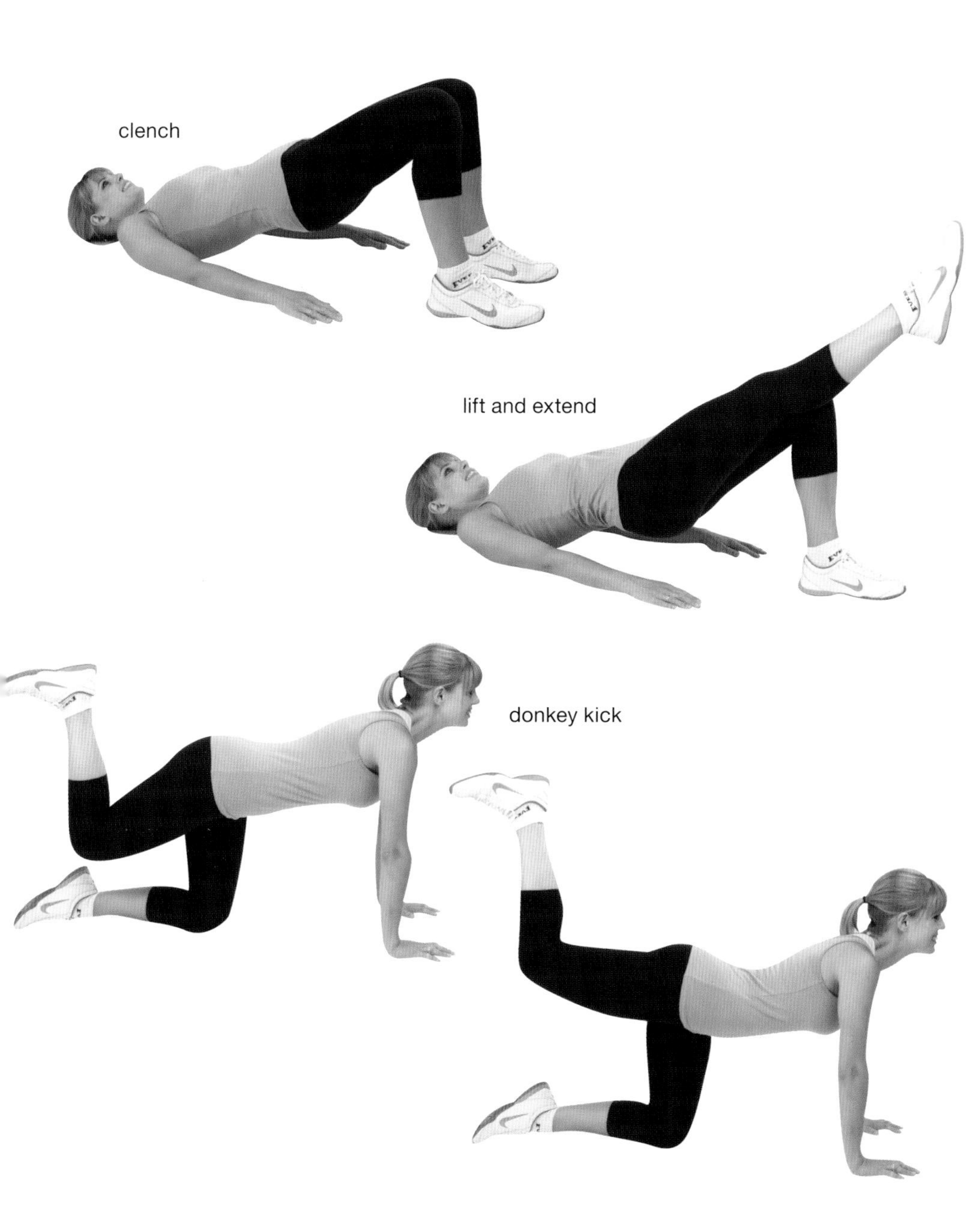
clench
lift and extend
donkey kick

side leg lift

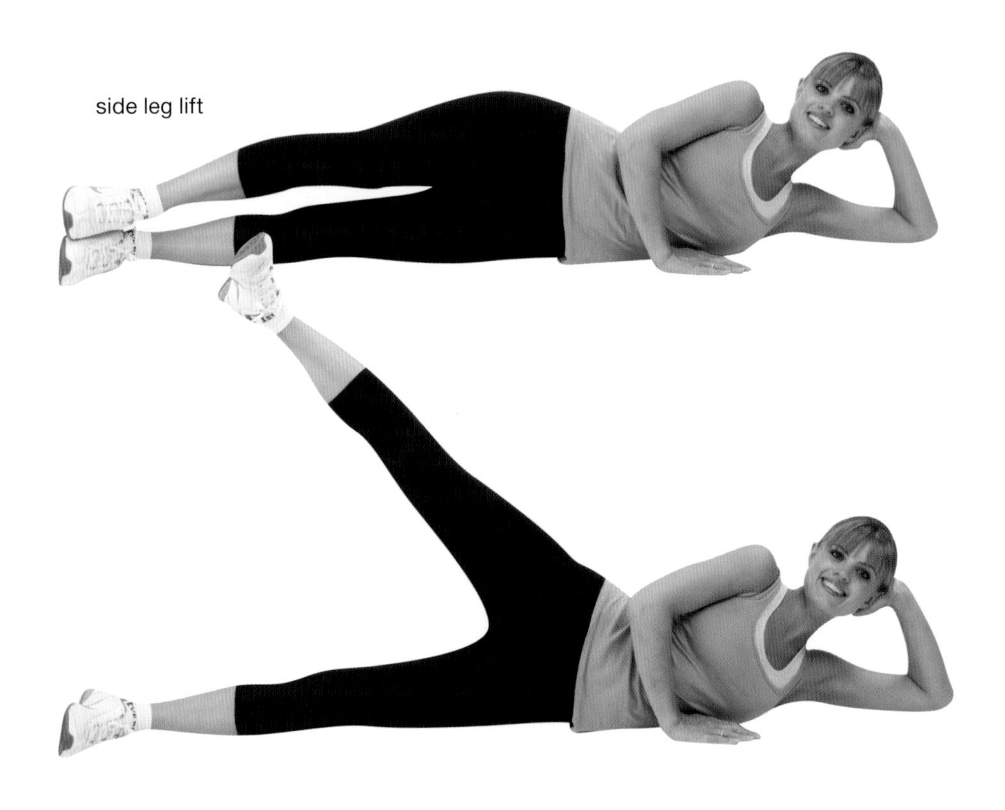

inner thigh lift

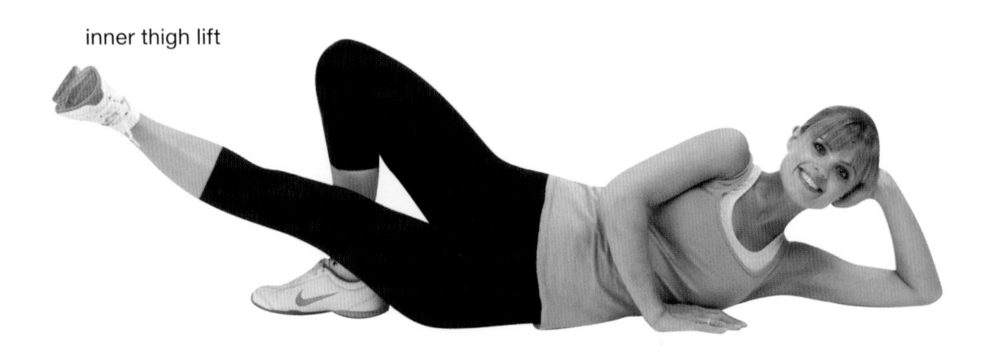

Toned thighs in ten

Work your outer and inner thighs with these leg lifts. Aim for control and effort – use your own body weight to provide resistance.

Side leg lifts

- Lie on one side in a straight line, with your elbow on the floor and your head resting on your hand
- Raise your upper leg into the air, keeping your leg straight. Flex your foot so it is facing forwards
- With control, lower your leg to the start position
- Repeat an equal number of times on both legs

Vary this by bringing the upper leg in front of you so it is almost at a 90-degree angle with the lower leg. With control, lift and lower for 10 reps. Repeat on the other side.

Inner thigh lifts

- Lie on one side, with one leg stretched out flat to the floor
- Bend the knee of the opposite leg and place the foot on the ground, behind the outstretched leg
- Raise your extended leg (foot flexed and facing forwards), keeping it straight, into the air. Feel the stretch along the inner thigh
- Lower the leg to the ground
- Repeat an equal number of times on both legs

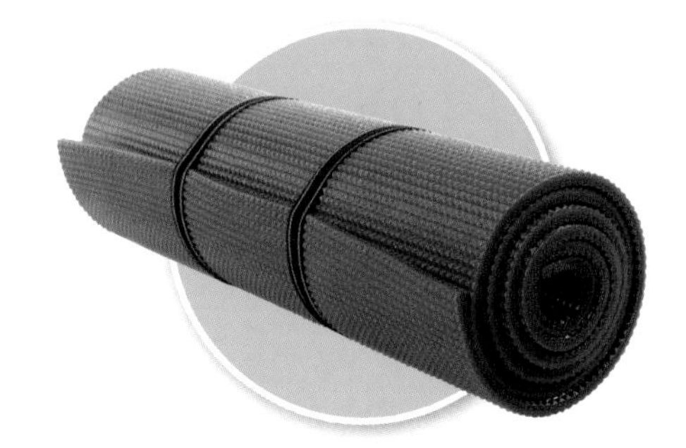

Abdominals

Strong abdominals are central to core strength, which supports all your workout activities.

Starter sit-up

- Lie on your back with your knees bent, feet flat on the floor
- Rest your hands on your thighs. Slowly slide them up your leg, towards your knees – lift with your abs. Lower with control
- Keep the lift and lower controlled

Do the starter sit-up before trying the full sit-up. Use your abdominals, not your lower back, to lift you.

Full sit-up

- Begin by lying on your back with your knees bent, making sure your feet are flat on the floor
- Bring your feet in towards your bottom and put your fingers behind your ears, looking upwards
- Bring your shoulders and upper body up towards your knees, elbows out

Lower body lifts

- Lie with your back flat on the floor with your arms by your sides, palms facing upwards
- Lift your legs in the air with feet pointing towards the ceiling

Bicycle

- Lie with your back on the floor. Lightly support your head with your fingers
- Using your stomach muscles, not your neck, bring your knees into your chest and lift your shoulder blades off the floor
- Bring your right elbow and left knee towards each other as you straighten out your right leg
- Switch sides, bringing your left elbow towards your right knee
- Continue the pedalling motion

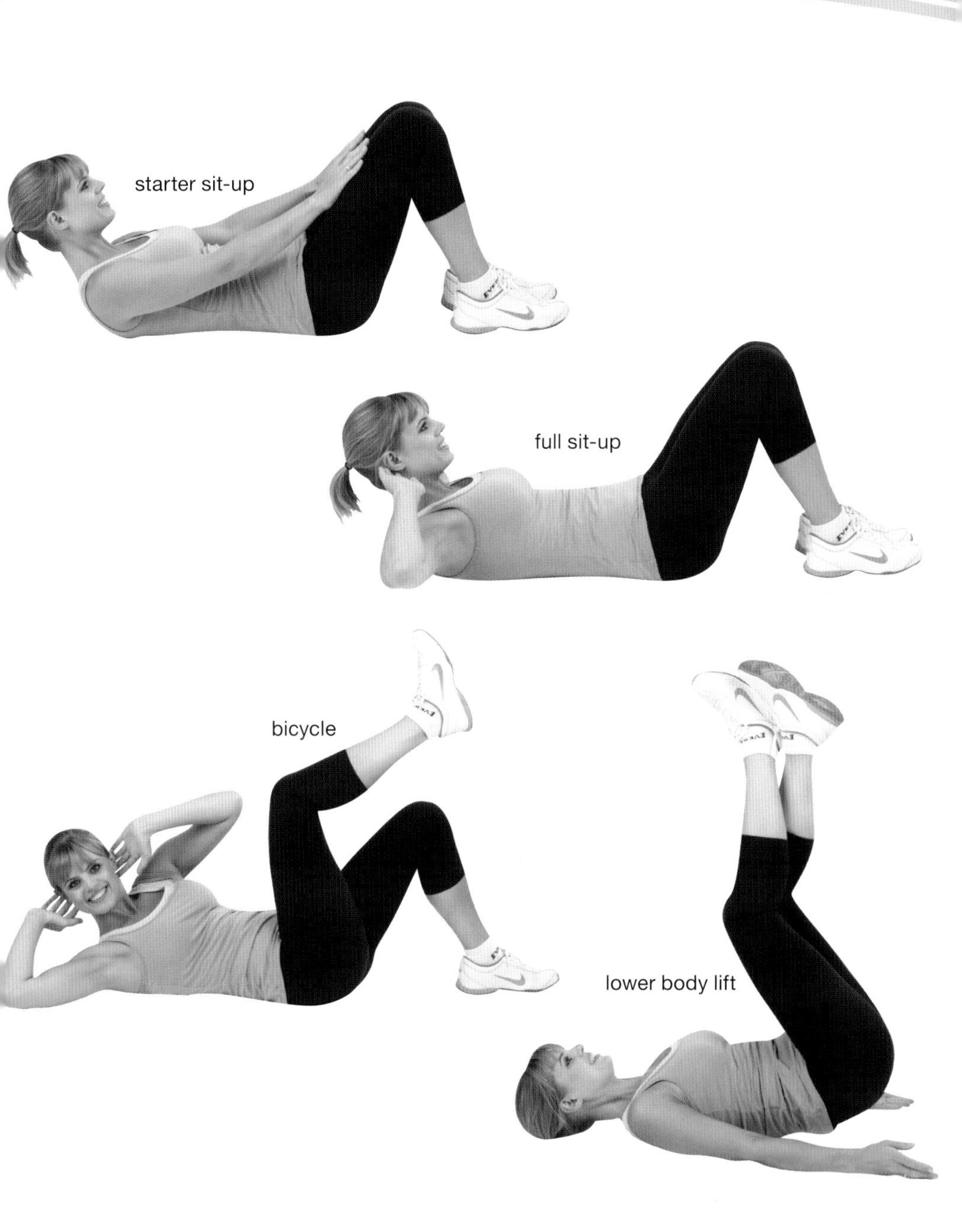
starter sit-up
full sit-up
bicycle
lower body lift

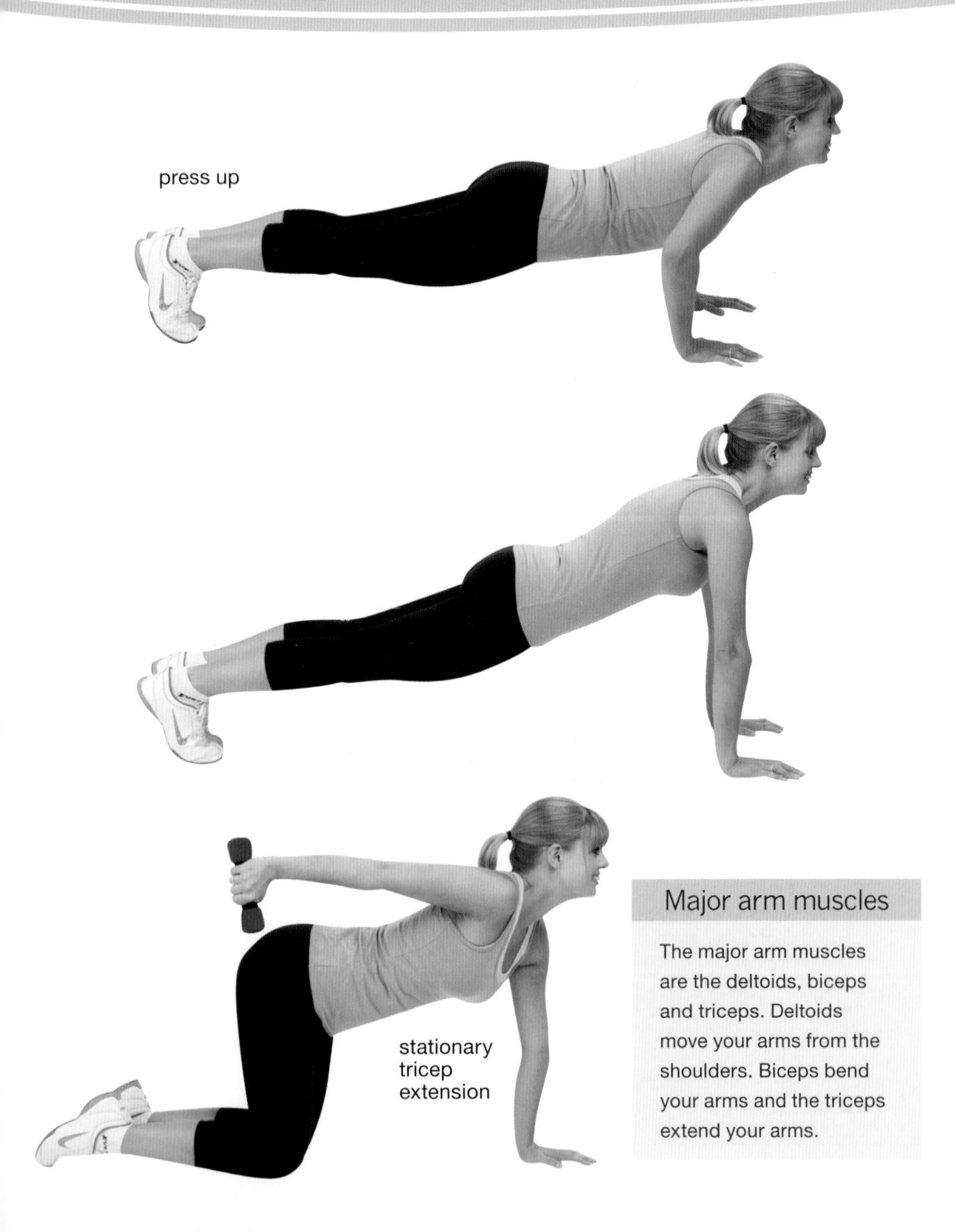

Major arm muscles

The major arm muscles are the deltoids, biceps and triceps. Deltoids move your arms from the shoulders. Biceps bend your arms and the triceps extend your arms.

Arms

As well as the tricep dip on page 60 and the weights exercises, these exercises will ensure your arms are toned. Incorporate the press up into your cardiovascular circuits session.

Press up

Lots of people do press ups, but incorrectly. Done properly, they are hard work and effective; done incorrectly they are ineffective.

- Place your hands underneath your shoulders with arms fully extended, palms flat and fingers facing forwards
- Keep your legs straight with your knees off the floor. Make sure your abs are tight, your back is not arched and your hips are not sinking
- Aim to lower yourself to about 5 cm (2 in) above the ground. Push back up. Do 10 reps

You can do this with your knees on the floor if you need to build up strength for the full press up.

Tricep extension

You can do this exercise when you are running at a moderate pace or walking at speed. Don't do it when you are sprinting.

- Lift your elbow behind you at a 90-degree angle. Straighten your lower arm, keeping your arm as strong as possible. Try not to let your arm drop
- Bring your lower arm back to the starting position and repeat 20 times. Swap sides and repeat

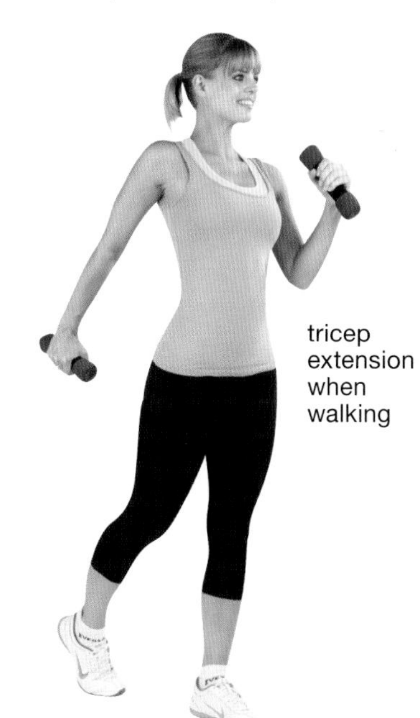

tricep extension when walking

Flex it up

Flexibility is how far your joints are able to move, which depends on the elasticity of your muscles. It's often left out from a workout or from an exercise regime because it doesn't raise a sweat. However, make it part of your fast fitness programme and you will see and feel the benefits.

Warm your body up with some rotations (slowly circle your ankles, lower leg, arms, neck) and march up and down or jog gently. Then incorporate these stretches into your warm-up or cool-down.

Tricep stretch

- Bend your elbow and lower your hand behind your back
- Hold your arm behind the elbow and feel the stretch in your tricep

Shoulder stretch

- Hold your arm across your chest, pressing on the upper arm with your free hand

Butterfly

This works inner thighs, knees and hips.

- Sit down with the soles of your feet together
- Drop your knees towards the ground
- Use your forearms to gently push your knees toward the ground
- Lean forward from the hips

Sitting wide-legged forward bend

This works the outer and inner thigh, hips and lower back.

- On the floor, with your legs wide, gently bring your upper body forwards from your hips, with your arms outstretched

Knees to chest

- Lie on your back with your knees bent. Hold the tops of your knees and pull them to your chest

Smooth stretches

It's ok to feel a mild pull when stretching, but it's not ok to feel pain. Stretches need to be smooth – not sudden, jerky movements. Hold each stretch for ten seconds.

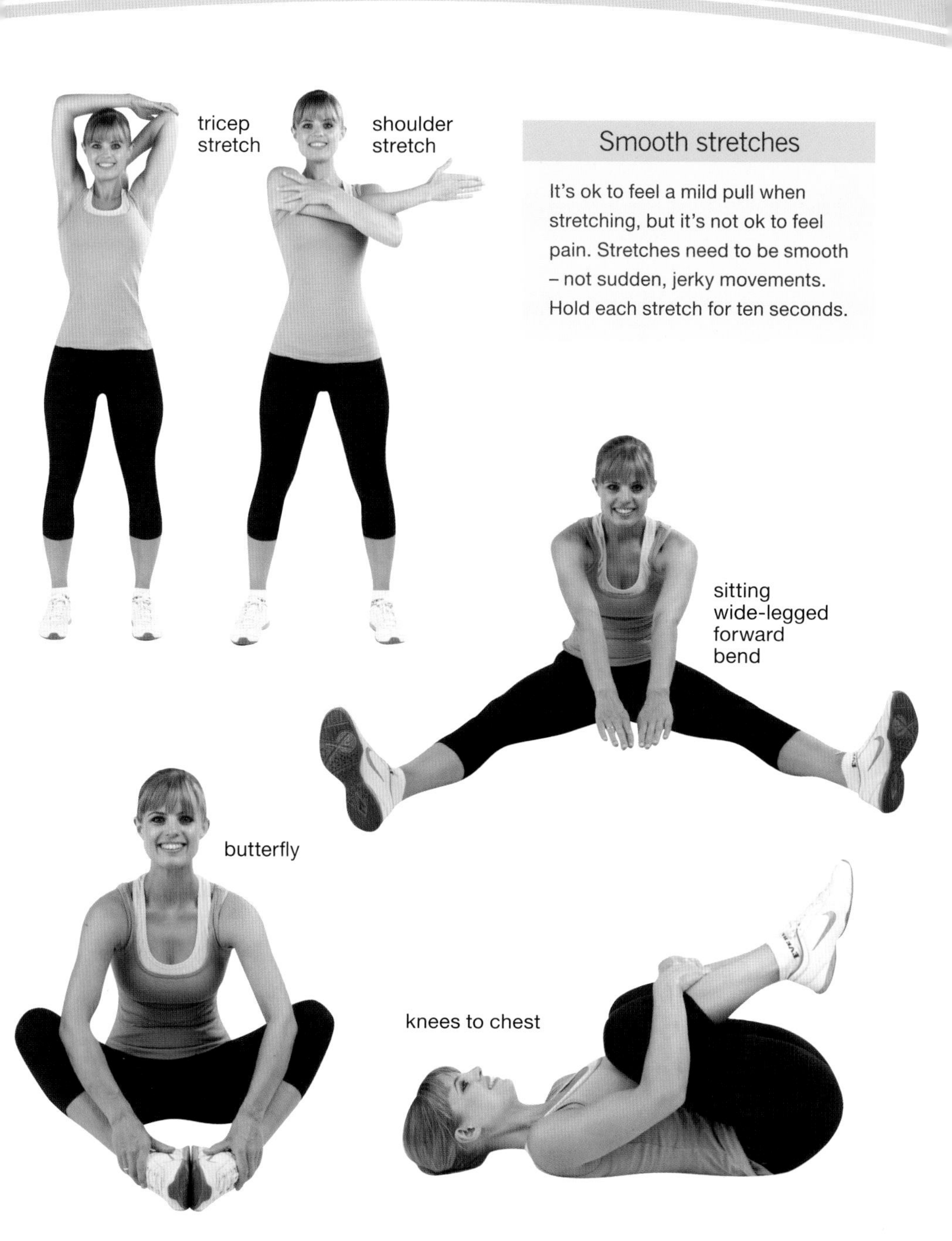

Kickbox

Kickboxing is a great way to work out. It's high intensity, can be done in your own home, and is a great workout in under ten minutes.

Fighting stance

This is your starting position. Stagger your feet – stand with one foot slightly in front of the other, back heel slightly raised. Keep your fists raised, near your jawline.

Jab

- With your right foot forwards, pull your right arm back
- Rotate from the right hip
- Shoot your arm forwards in a short straight punch
- Pull your arm back with control
- Repeat on the other side

Cross

- From your fighting stance with your right foot forwards, turn your left foot, hip and knee to the right as you punch forwards with your left hand
- Pull back with control
- Repeat on the other side

Side kick

- Stand in fighting stance, right foot forwards
- Turn your hips to the left
- Lift your right leg and with a flexed foot, push through your heel to kick your leg out
- Lean your upper body to the left
- Pull back with control
- Repeat on the other side

Two workouts in one

Kickboxing is both an aerobic and anaerobic workout. The high-intensity, fast movements give your heart and lungs a workout. Your muscles are tested too by the kicking and jabbing, and also by maintaining the fighting stance position.

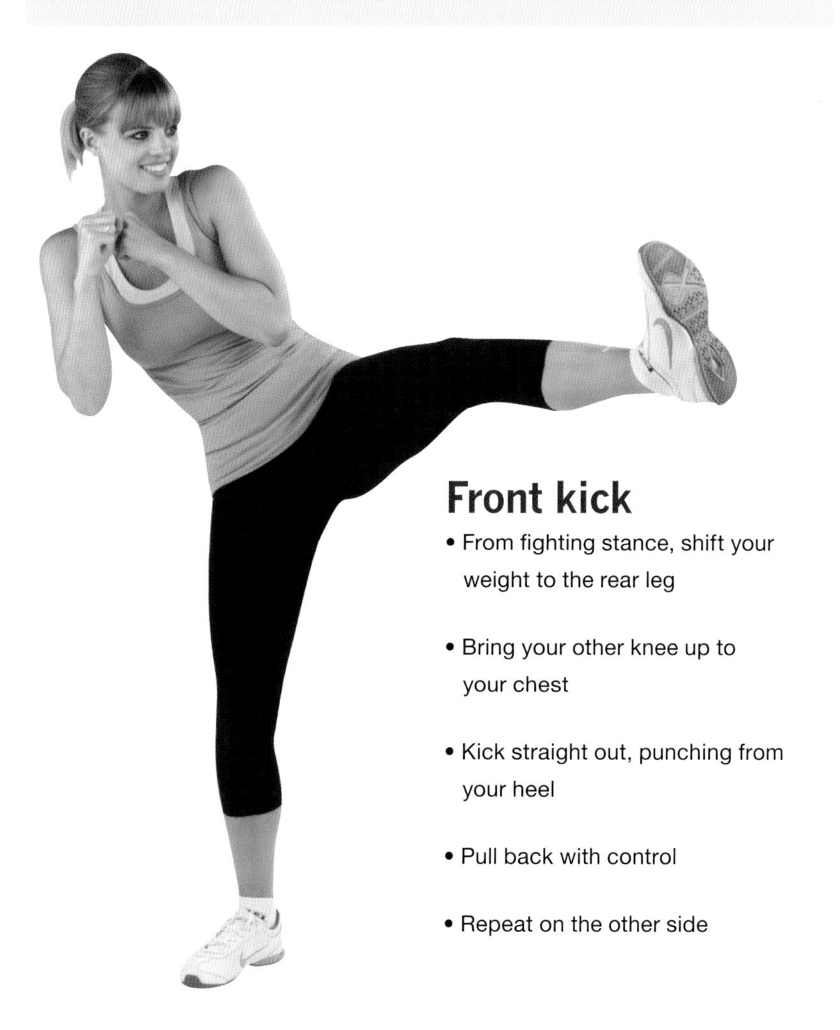

Front kick

- From fighting stance, shift your weight to the rear leg
- Bring your other knee up to your chest
- Kick straight out, punching from your heel
- Pull back with control
- Repeat on the other side

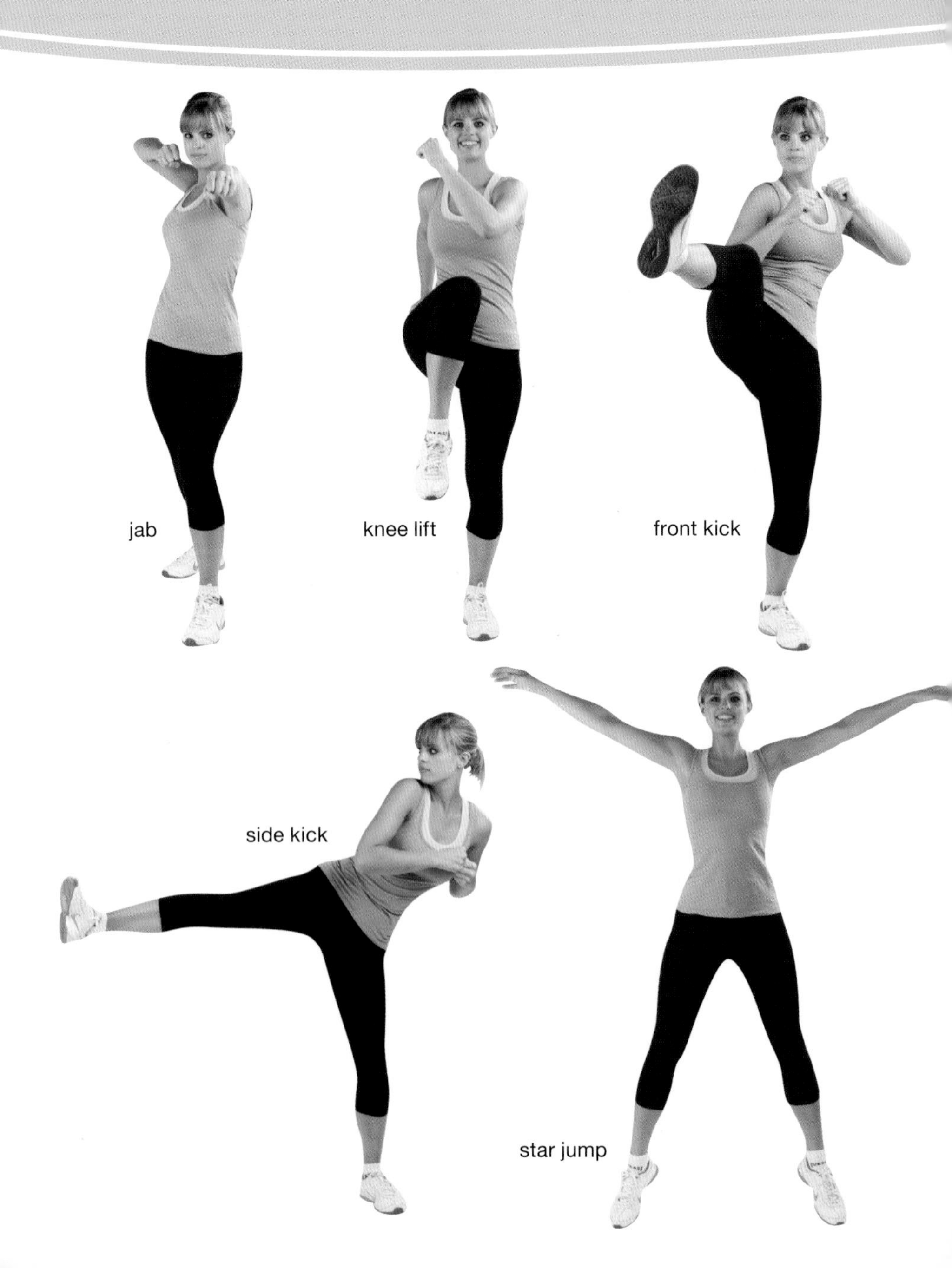
jab
knee lift
front kick
side kick
star jump

The following routines will work you at fever pitch. Keep your abs tight.

Warm up

March on the spot. Start with your knees low, and increase the intensity with a higher knee lift. Add in your arms, pumping them. Next, step from side to side, swinging your arms.

A: Total time 6 minutes

2 minute warm-up

30 seconds jabs on both sides

30 seconds crosses, both sides

2 minute cool-down and stretch out

B: Total time 4 minutes 10 seconds

2 minute warm-up

40 seconds front kicks

60 seconds recovery (marching)

50 seconds side kicks

70 seconds recovery

30 seconds jabs

2 minute cool-down and stretch out

C: Total time 13 minutes 20 seconds

2 minute warm-up

60 second sequence: 1 jab, 1 cross, 2 knee lifts (low and high) followed by 1 star jump. With the low knee lift, keep your knee bent and then fully extend it for the high knee lift. Turn to the other side on the star jump to repeat the sequence on the other leg

80 seconds recovery

Repeat 4 times

2 minute cool-down and stretch out

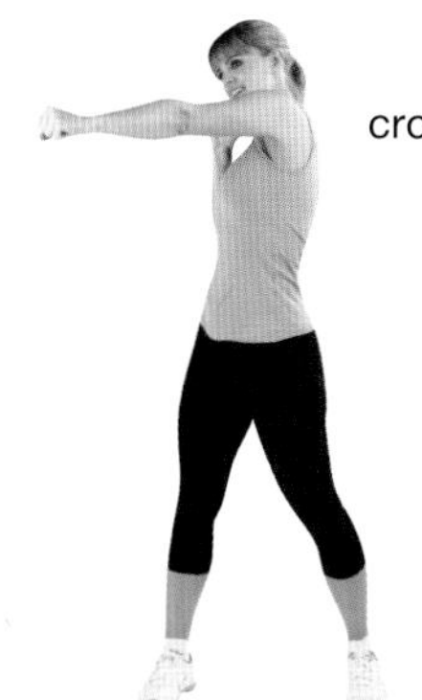

crosses

Moving Fast

Not keen on a run or cycle? How about a bounce on a trampoline, or some high-energy dancing to fast-paced music for ten minutes?

Dance it off

Warm up just as you would for any of the exercises and workouts in this book. Alternate your energised dance moves and jumps with some slower gentler moves that will allow your body to recover enough to raise the tempo for the next moves. Time your playlist to mix fast beats followed by slower tracks – that way you literally move to the music.

Incorporate some star jumps and squats for maximum effect.

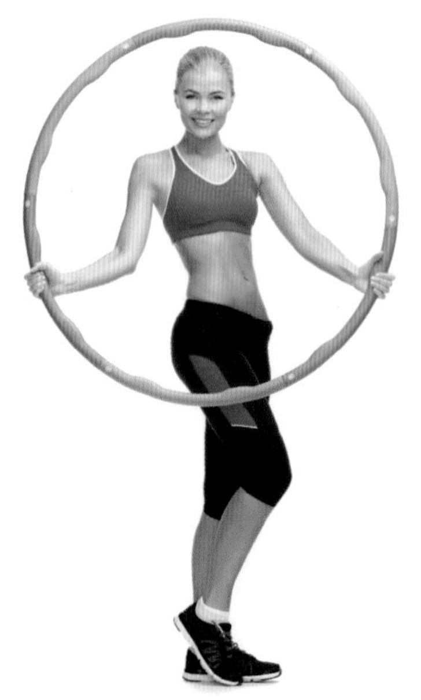

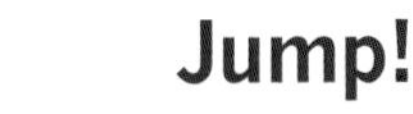

Jump!

If you have access to a mini trampoline (or a regular-sized one) then start jumping. Trampolines are great for a cardio workout. Make sure the trampoline is secure. You need to be careful when you are working at high intensity – falling off is painful and not a great look!

Jog, sprint (on the spot), bounce, star jump or squat – you can do any of these moves on a trampoline. Make sure you add in recovery time with some gentle bouncing.

Twist

Remember hula hoops? Well, they are pretty good for a workout. Like skipping, it takes practice, but once you've got the hang of it, make it harder by adding in different moves.

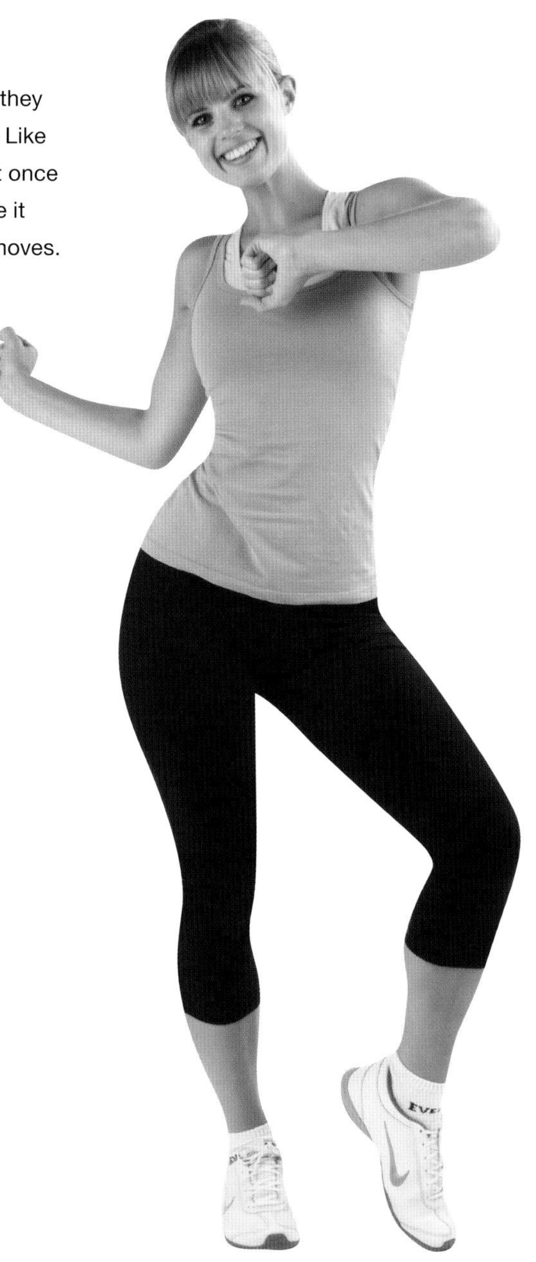

Dance smart!

Dancing is good for your brain. Freestyle dancing can even prevent memory loss because the brain has to keep rewiring its neural pathways.

Mix It Up

Keep your workout interesting by mixing up different activities. This is great fun if you can do it with a friend or exercise buddy.

Plan

With all workouts, it's best to have an idea of what you are going to cover. Ten minutes isn't long, and you won't get your high intensity from standing and wondering what to do next!

Cycle and run

Mix cycling with running. Depending on where you are working out, you might need to lock up your bike during your recovery before you start your high intensity run.

Run and circuits

If you are out in the park, it's easy to combine running with circuits. Find a park bench and do 30 step ups.

Run and kick

Run, recover, kickbox, recover and run.

Weights and run

Drop your weights on the ground, along with your water, and run for 30 seconds. Jog back to retrieve your weights and work out with them for one minute. Keep it going until you have worked out completely.

Swim and kick

Mix some kickboxing moves into your swimming plan – keeping it fresh helps you keep motivated.

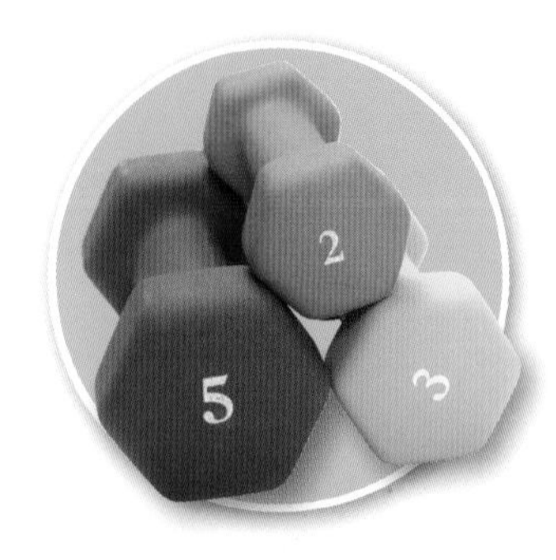

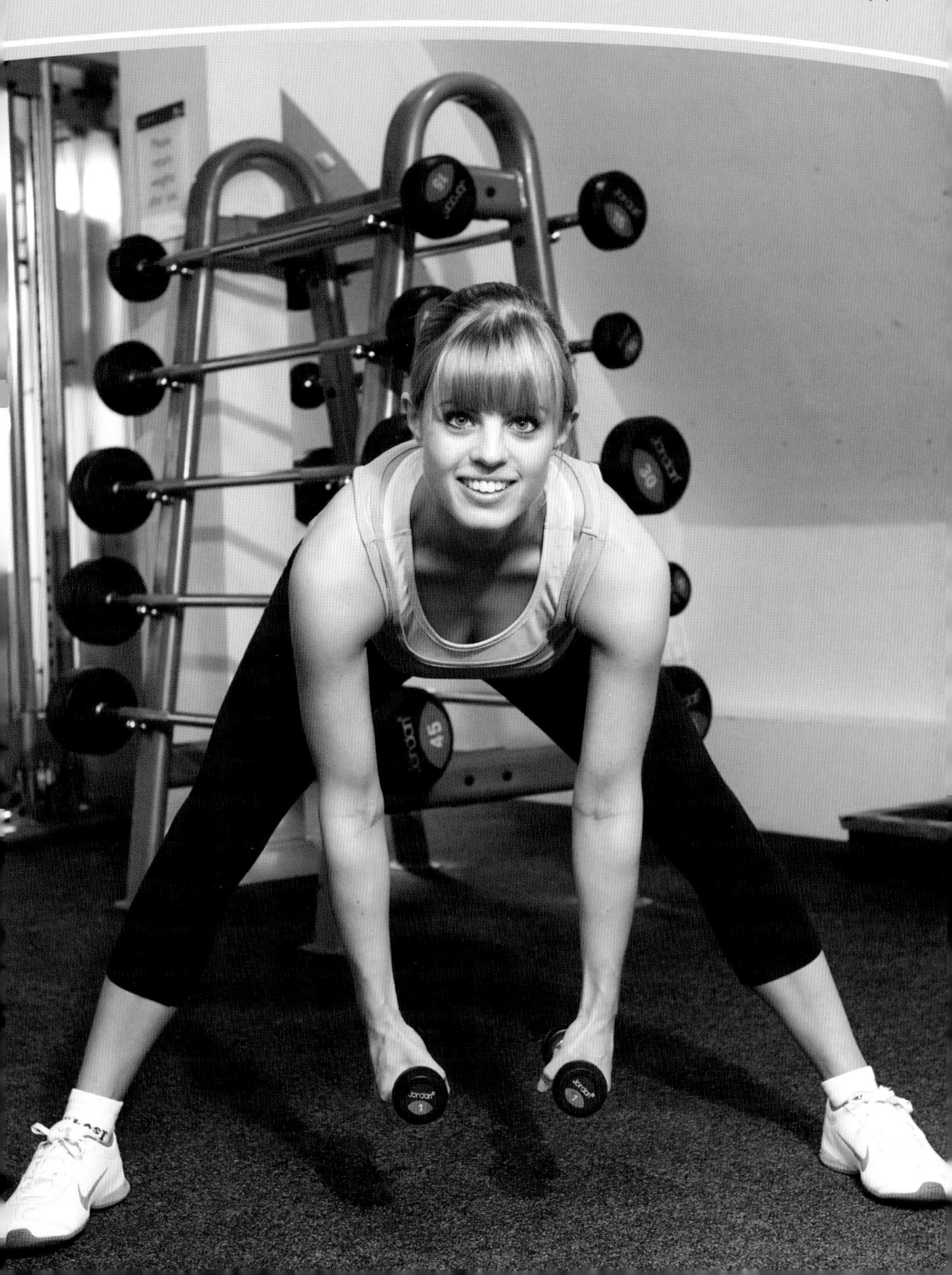
Jordan
45
30

Make It Work

Home, work and play – there doesn't seem to be enough time to do everything. Fast fitness exercises and routines fit into your life, making it easier.

Work out at work. You may not be able to sprint, cycle or swim but you can work hard. Close the door if you can, and if not, find somewhere with a bit of space such as a car park (but not at busy times) where you can do some circuits.

Obviously you need to adapt the exercises and routine to your place of work. If you work in a library, it's not ideal to do star jumps on the floor above the quiet reading room, or if you work in a hospital it won't be safe to bound up the stairs curling your biceps as patients gingerly make their way down! If your place of work isn't any good, head outdoors – you can still train in the rain.

Can you make your journey to work part of your workout? If you walk to work, invest in a backpack and spend ten minutes of your walk getting fit fast. If you cycle, adapt your route so that you can cycle safely at speed along a track. If you drive to work or get public transport, leave the car a ten minute walk away or get off before your stop and speed walk instead. You will need a backpack instead of holding on to a bag which would restrict the efficiency of your swing and stride.

No shower at work? Take a spare set of clothes, some deodorant or body spray and freshen up in the bathrooms.

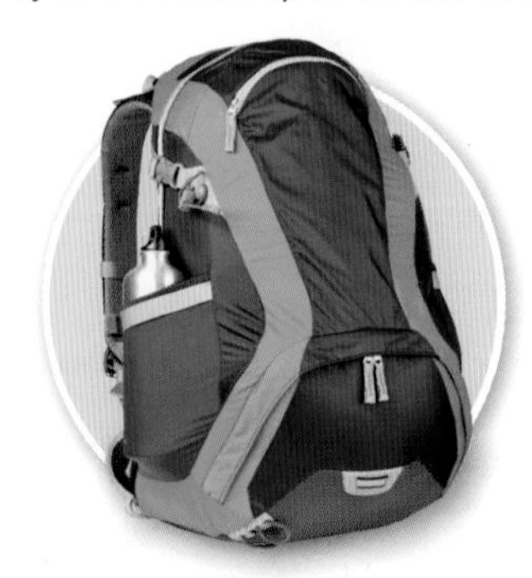

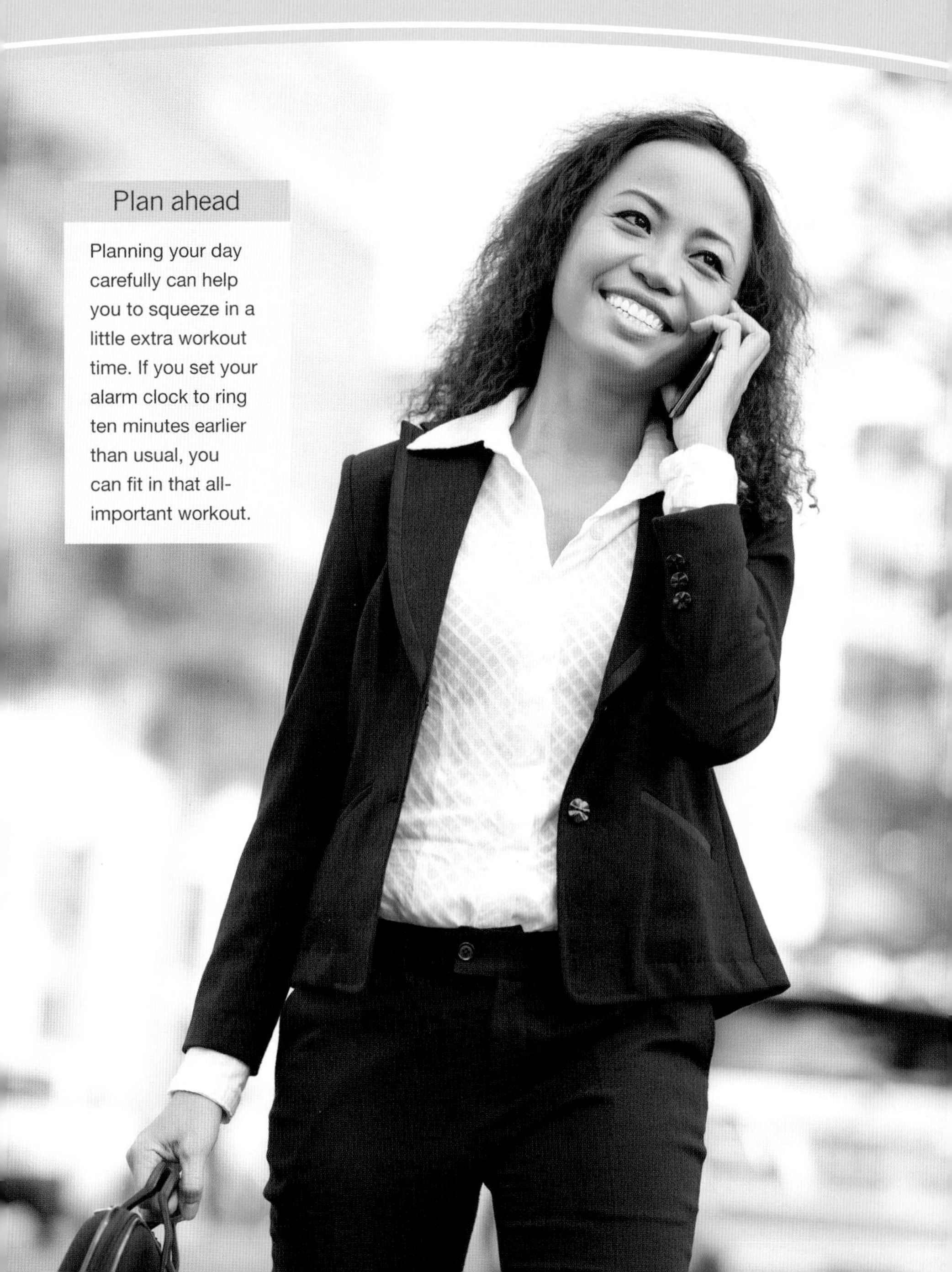

Plan ahead

Planning your day carefully can help you to squeeze in a little extra workout time. If you set your alarm clock to ring ten minutes earlier than usual, you can fit in that all-important workout.

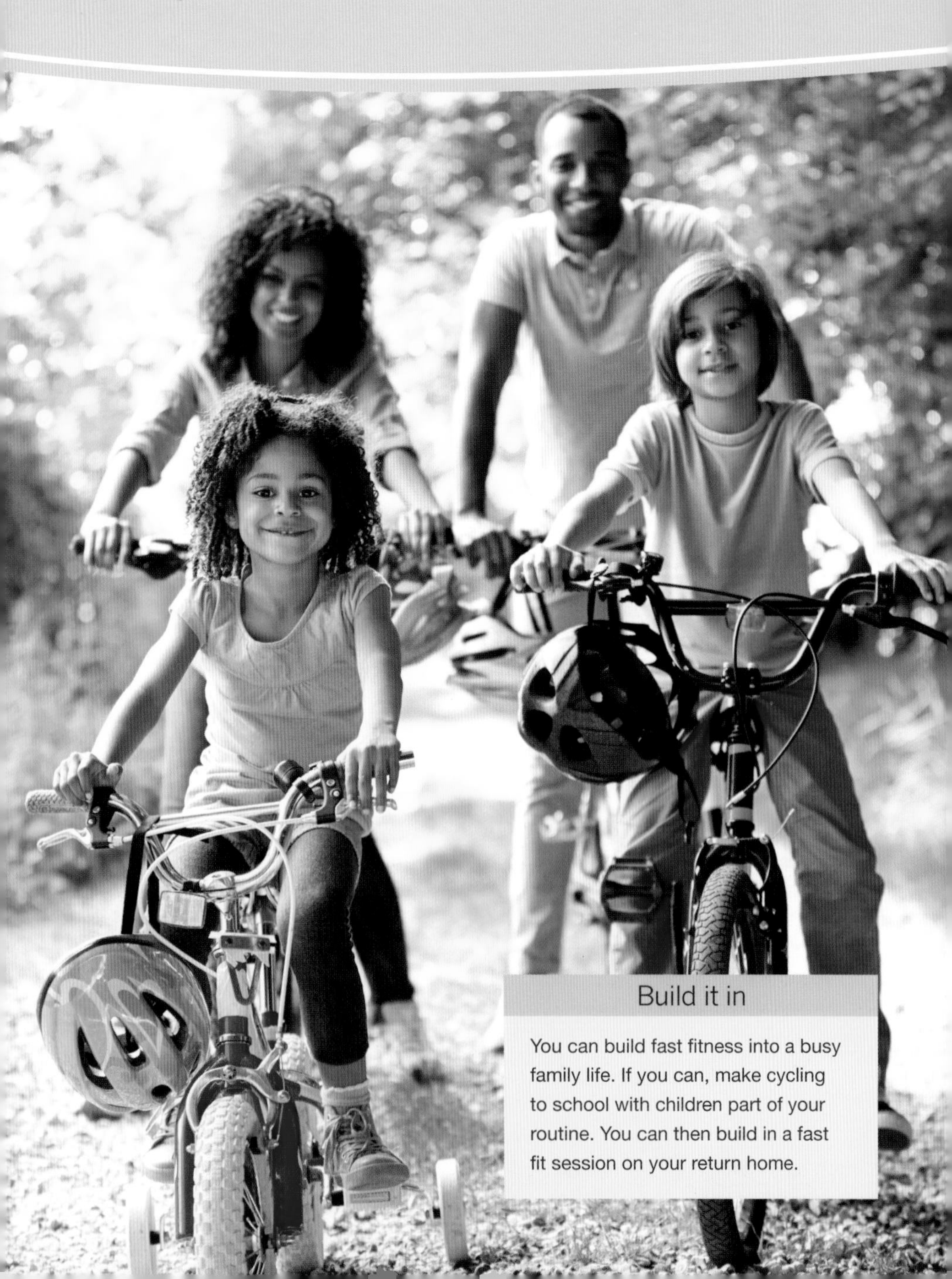

Build it in

You can build fast fitness into a busy family life. If you can, make cycling to school with children part of your routine. You can then build in a fast fit session on your return home.

Don't worry about what other people think, whether you're at work or in the park – they probably wish they had your motivation. See if there is someone who can be an exercise buddy with whom you can nip out for ten minutes. Working out with someone else helps keep up momentum – it's harder to make excuses when someone else is ready to go.

Kickboxing is good to do at work or after a difficult day. It gets rid of a lot of energy and tension, and you can also let go of pent-up aggression by imagining you are sparring with a real- life opponent.

Look around the office or workplace for sturdy chairs or suitable boxes. Do some tricep dips (see page 60) or some step ups (just make sure you won't slip, the furniture is stable and at the correct height).

Kids on holiday?

Kickbox at home. Teach the kids some moves (but be aware that this exercise pattern is not for children – let children have fun with exercise and do as much as they can enjoy in their own time and way). Ask the kids to time you – after all, the durations are so short that they won't get bored and leave you jabbing and hooking for hours!

Take older kids swimming. While they splash about or whizz down the water slide, you can get in a couple of serious laps and then join them to splash around as part of your recovery! Dancing at home is fun and can be a great quick workout. Turn up the volume and get moving. Remember, your workout should fit around your lifestyle, so these short bursts of exercise are great for times like these.

Take it to the park

Parks are perfect for high intensity exercise. You could sprint and recover, step up (on a bench) and recover or lunge and recover. Try tricep dips on a bench – all the equipment you need is in the park, it takes ten minutes and you're getting fresh air.

Fast Fit Food

Feed your body – food is the fuel that gives you energy. Similarly, not eating enough will leave your body craving nutrition, and the intense workouts will put a strain on your physical health.

Top tips

- After a meal, wait for a couple of hours before you exercise
- If you feel a bit jelly-like after your workout, keep a healthy snack in your bag such as a banana
- A cup of hot water with a slice of lemon is a wonderfully cleansing way to start the day
- If you want to get in your fast fitness very early in the morning, have your breakfast afterwards
- Plan in your meals and snacks – that way you are less likely to grab a packet of crisps or some chocolate
- Drink plenty of water
- Choose wholegrain foods, such as wholegrain bread, rather than refined, processed foods
- Watch out for added sugar, salt and fat in processed foods. Avoid refined foods which have been processed and had most of their natural goodness removed

The good and the bad

There are always headlines proclaiming that for example, bananas are the worst food you can eat, a blueberry will transform your life and running makes you fat. Take it all with a pinch of salt. Bananas are an excellent source of energy; blueberries are packed with nutrients but they won't make your life perfect; and running won't make you fat.

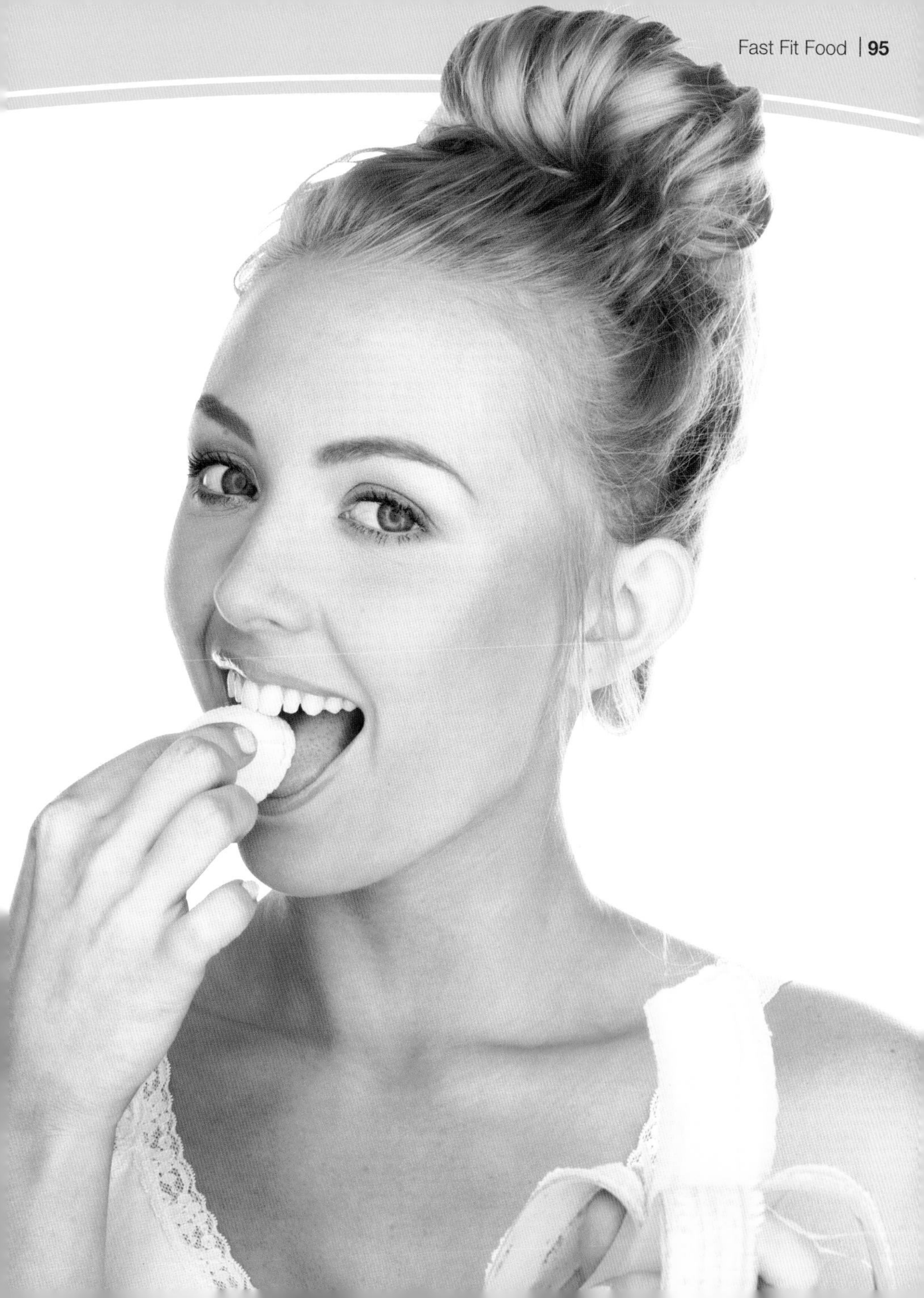

What's best?

There are so many diets and programmes for weight loss, but the key is moderation and making sure that your body is getting the nutrients it needs for best performance. Choose a balanced diet with regular meals and regular portions (certainly not super-sized ones) and you will get the vitamins and minerals you need to keep your body fighting fit.

A fatty fix

Fats matter because some of them help the body absorb certain nutrients and provide essential fatty acids. Less important fats are the ones we often eat too many of – these are the saturated fats in foods such as fatty meats and cheese.

Most saturated fats come from dairy and animal products (apart from palm and coconut oils). Too many saturated fats are linked to raising the risk of cardiovascular disease – the exact opposite of what you are aiming for with fast fitness. Avoid saturated fats where possible.

Aim to eat plenty of unsaturated fats found in oily fish (salmon, sardines and mackerel), nuts and seeds.

Sugar

Fizzy drinks contain spoons and spoons of sugar. Cut back as much as you can on sugar – it provides empty calories, and there is already lots of natural sugar in the healthy foods we eat before we start sprinkling sugar in coffee and tea.

Protein

If you are very active you need to eat lots of protein. Chicken, fish, lean red meat and low-fat dairy foods are all good sources of protein. Snack on nuts and seeds rather than biscuits or chocolates.

Carbohydrates

These get a mixed press, but carbohydrates provide energy for your body's work. There are three types of carbohydrates: sugar, starch and fibre. Starchy foods provide a slow release of energy throughout the day. In the winter, a bowl of porridge oats is perfect for breakfast.

Fresh fruit and veg

Think multicoloured – the more colour you can get into your diet (natural colours, not E numbers), the better. Choose carrots, tomatoes, broccoli, oranges, beetroot, watercress, peppers, blueberries and more.

Liquid

Drink water when you are thirsty. It's important not to get dehydrated, but it is important also not to drink too much as this can also be dangerous.

And talking of drinking: alcohol – it's not a good idea to exercise at high intensity if you have had a heavy night out and drunk too much. You will be dehydrated and working out at high intensity will put a strain on your body. Alcohol is also packed with empty calories.

Eat a rainbow!

A rainbow diet – one full of colours – will provide your body with the range of nutrients that it needs.

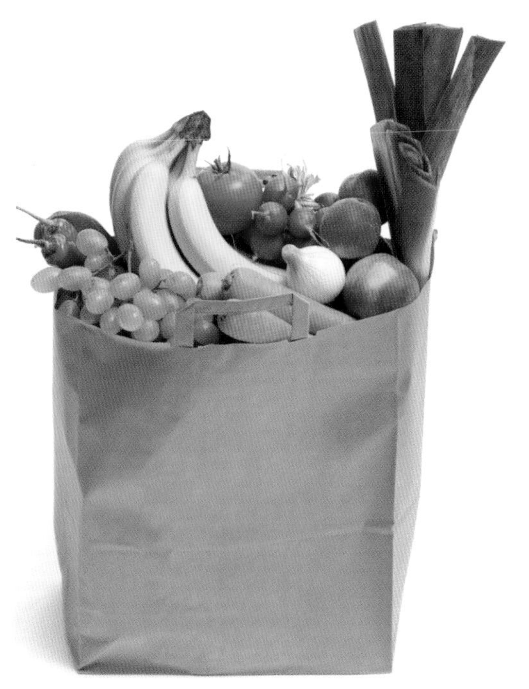

Calorie Check

Calories are a measure of the amount of energy in food. The more physical activity you do, the more energy (calories) you use.

It's useful to know roughly how many calories are in particular foods, and how many calories you use up through different exercises. But it's only part of the picture. Aim to think about balancing a healthy eating pattern with a vigorous and sustained exercise programme, rather than counting the calories of every mouthful or every minute of exercise.

The following is a rough guide to the number of calories used during exercise. The amount used will depend on your age, weight, sex and the intensity of the exercise. There are some good online calculators and phone apps to give you a more tailored figure. Remember, with fast fitness, your body still burns calories long after you finish exercising.

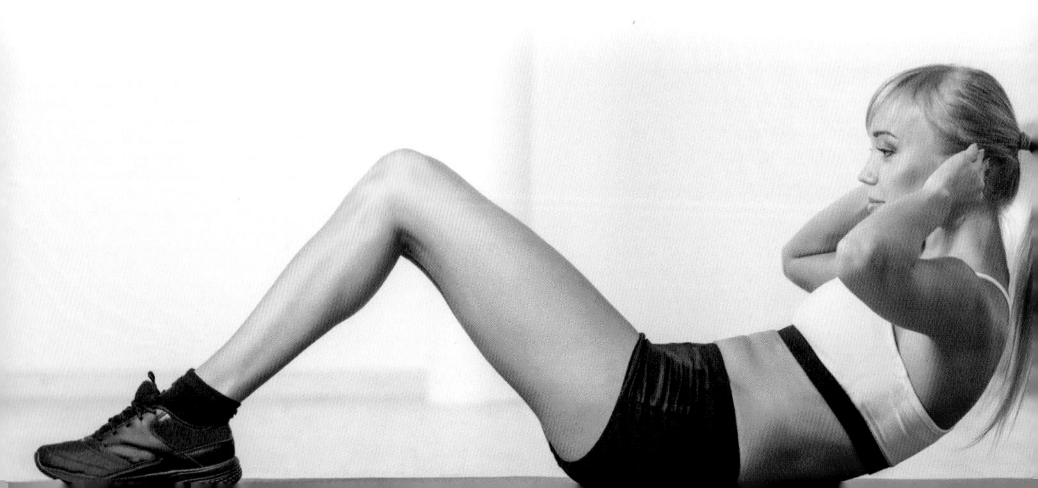

Activity	Calories burned per hour by an individual weighing: 58 kg (9 st 4 lb)	70 kg (11 st 1 lb)	81 kg (12 st 12 lb)
Badminton	266	317	368
Canoeing, rowing, vigorous	708	844	981
Circuit training, minimal rest	472	563	654
Cycling, 19–22 kph, moderate	472	563	654
Cycling, 22–25 kph, vigorous	590	704	817
Cycling, 25–30 kph, very fast, racing	708	844	981
Football or baseball, playing catch	148	176	204
Gardening, general	236	281	327
Frisbee playing, general	177	211	245
Housework, vigorous	236	281	327
Skipping, fast	708	844	981
Skipping, moderate	590	704	817
Running, 8 kph	472	563	654
Running, 11 kph	679	809	940
Running, 17 kph	1062	1267	1471
Running up stairs	885	1056	1226
Stationary cycling, light	325	387	449
Stationary cycling, moderate	413	493	572
Stationary cycling, vigorous	620	739	858
Stationary cycling, very vigorous	738	880	1022
Swimming backstroke	413	493	572
Swimming breaststroke	590	704	817
Swimming butterfly	649	774	899
Swimming laps, freestyle, fast	590	704	817
Swimming laps, freestyle, slow	413	493	572
Swimming leisurely, not laps	354	422	490
Swimming sidestroke	472	563	654
Swimming, treading water, fast	590	704	817
Swimming, treading water, moderate	236	281	327
Table tennis, ping pong	236	281	327
Trampoline	207	246	286
Walk/run, playing, moderate	236	281	327
Walk/run, playing, vigorous	295	352	409
Walking 3 kph, slow	148	176	204
Walking 5 kph, moderate	195	232	270
Walking 6 kph, brisk pace	224	267	311
Walking 5.5 kph, uphill	354	422	490
Walking 6.5 kph, very brisk	295	352	409
Walking 7 kph	372	443	515
Walking 8 kph	472	563	654

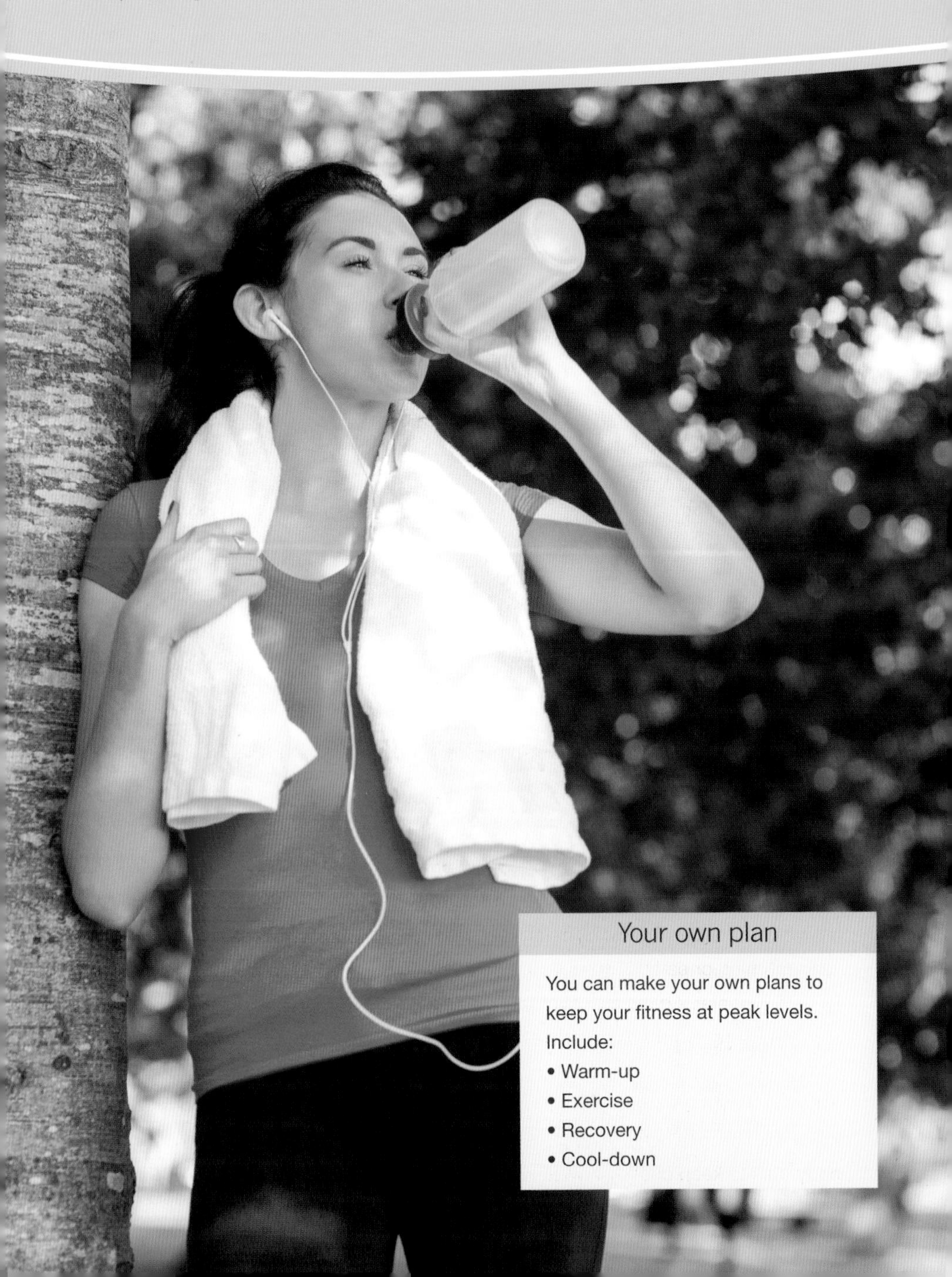

Your own plan

You can make your own plans to keep your fitness at peak levels. Include:

- Warm-up
- Exercise
- Recovery
- Cool-down

Exercise Plans

All of the exercise plans provided are guides to get you started. They are varied to cater for beginners and intermediate. Please note, beginner does not mean that you are new to exercise; it means you already have a good level of fitness.

The plans on the following pages are based on working out at high intensity, three times a week.

Each plan has a minimum two-minute warm-up and cool-down. Do not do less than this.

Weather wise

Do not work out at high intensity when it is very hot or very humid. Aim for early morning or early evening instead when it is cooler. Adapt your exercise plan to ensure you do not become dehydrated or suffer from heatstroke or exhaustion. Make sure you drink more water than usual when it is hot. The body tries to keep cool by sweating more, which draws out more of the water in your body. This can leave you dehydrated.

When it is cold and/or wet, you need to be more careful of slipping when running or cycling. When it is cold, take a jumper or fleece with you to wear during your warm-up and cool-down. Make sure you warm up properly as your joints and muscles will literally need warming up.

Challenge yourself

Whether you follow the plans on pages 102–111 or devise your own workout programme, be honest with yourself. If your exercise regime is getting easy, make it harder. If it is so hard that you are giving up, adapt it to make it work. Add in challenges, change the types of exercise you are doing, and keep it fresh. That way your motivation is more likely to keep you going on to better health and better fitness.

Week 1
Starting Out

Day 1

Cycle
3 minute warm-up
20 seconds cycle (high intensity)
80 seconds recovery
Repeat 2 times
3 minute cool-down and stretch out

Day 3

Run
3 minute warm-up
20 seconds run (high intensity)
80 seconds recovery
Repeat 2 times
2 minute cool-down and stretch out

Day 5

Swim
3 minute warm-up
20 seconds swim (high intensity)
80 seconds recovery
Repeat 2 times
2 minute cool-down and stretch out

Week 1 Intermediate

Day 1

Cycle
2 minute warm-up
30 seconds cycle (high intensity)
80 seconds recovery
Repeat 2 times
2 minute cool-down and stretch out

Day 3

Run
2 minute warm-up
40 seconds run (high intensity)
80 seconds recovery
Repeat 3 times
2 minute cool-down and stretch out

Day 5

Swim
3 minute warm-up
40 seconds swim (high intensity)
80 seconds recovery
Repeat 3 times
2 minute cool-down and stretch out

Week 2 Starting Out

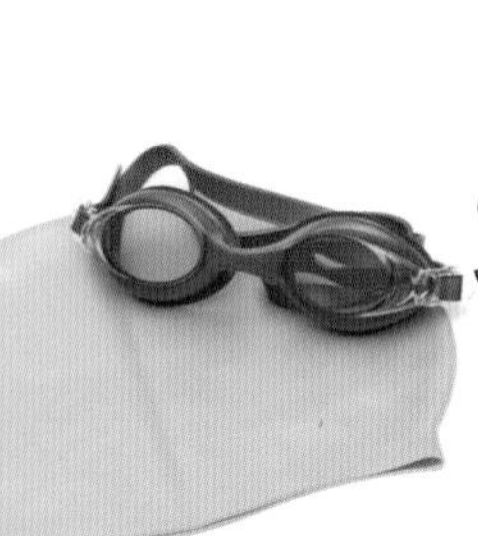

Day 1	**Walk** 4 minute warm-up 60 seconds walk (high intensity) 2 minute recovery Repeat 3 times 2 minute cool-down and stretch out
Day 3	**Swim (change your stroke)** 4 minute warm-up 30 seconds swim 60 seconds recovery Repeat 3 times 2 minute cool-down and stretch out
Day 5	**Kickbox** 3 minute warm-up 40 seconds front kicks 60 seconds recovery (marching) 50 seconds side kicks 70 second recovery 30 seconds jabs 2 minute cool-down and stretch out

Week 2 Intermediate

Day 1

Walk
4 minute warm-up
60 seconds walk (high intensity)
2 minute recovery
Repeat 4 times
2 minute cool-down and stretch out

Day 3

Swim (change your stroke)
4 minute warm-up
40 seconds swim
60 seconds recovery
Repeat 4 times
2 minute cool-down and stretch out

Day 5

Kickbox
3 minute warm-up
60 seconds: jab, cross, knee lifts (low and high), star jump (both sides of body)
80 seconds recovery
Repeat 4 times
2 minute cool-down and stretch out

Week 3
Starting Out

Day 1

Cycle
2 minute warm-up
30 seconds cycle (high intensity)
80 seconds recovery
Repeat 2 times
2 minute cool-down and stretch out

Day 3

Run
2 minute warm-up
30 seconds run (high intensity)
90 seconds recovery
Repeat 3 times
2 minute cool-down and stretch out

Day 5

Circuits
3 minute warm-up
30 seconds skip
40 seconds recover
30 seconds lunge (both legs)
30 seconds recovery
30 seconds tricep dips
2 minute cool-down and stretch out

Week 3 Intermediate

Day 1

Cycle
2 minute warm-up
40 seconds cycle (high intensity)
80 seconds recovery
Repeat 2 times
2 minute cool-down and stretch out

Day 3

Run uphill
2 minute warm-up
40 seconds run (high intensity)
90 seconds recovery
Repeat 3 times
2 minute cool-down and stretch out

Day 5

Circuits
3 minute warm-up
30 seconds squats
40 seconds recovery
30 seconds knee lifts with weights
40 seconds recovery
40 seconds press ups
40 seconds recovery
40 seconds lunge with single arm rows
2 minute cool-down and stretch out

Week 4
Starting Out

Day 1

Walk
4 minute warm-up
2 minutes walk (high intensity)
2 minute recovery
Repeat 4 times
2 minute cool-down and stretch out

Day 3

Cycle
2 minute warm-up
30 seconds cycle (high intensity)
60 seconds recovery
Repeat 3 times
2 minute cool-down and stretch out

Day 5

Swim
4 minute warm-up
40 seconds swim
60 seconds recovery
Repeat 3 times
2 minute cool-down and stretch out

Week 4 Intermediate

Day 1

Walk Uphill
4 minute warm-up
1 minute walk (high intensity)
2 minute recovery
2 minutes walk (high intensity)
2 minutes recovery
2 minutes walk (high intensity)
2 minute cool-down and stretch out

Day 3

Cycle Uphill
2 minute warm-up
40 seconds cycle (high intensity)
60 seconds recovery
Repeat 3 times
2 minute cool-down and stretch out

Day 5

Swim
4 minute warm-up
60 seconds swim
Repeat 5 times
2 minute cool-down and stretch out

Week 5
Starting Out

Day 1

Cycle
2 minute warm-up
40 seconds cycle (high intensity)
60 seconds recovery
Repeat 3 times
2 minute cool-down and stretch out

Day 3

Run Uphill
4 minute warm-up
40 seconds run (high intensity)
2 minutes recovery
Repeat 3 times
2 minute cool-down and stretch out

Day 5

Circuits
3 minute warm-up
30 seconds squats
60 seconds recovery
30 seconds press ups
60 seconds recovery
60 seconds leg lifts
60 seconds recovery
30 seconds plank
2 minute cool-down and stretch out

Week 5 Intermediate

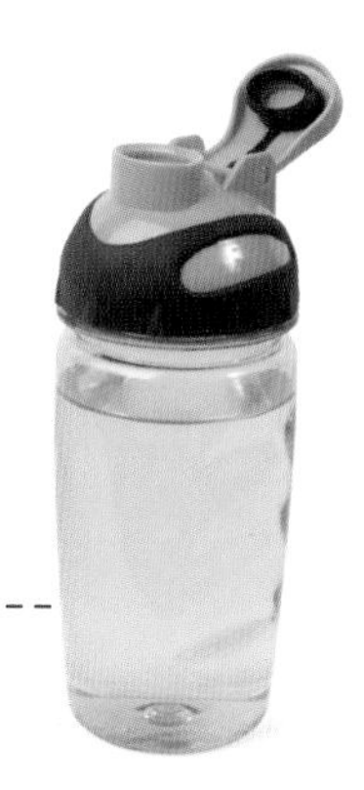

Day 1

Cycle
2 minute warm-up
60 seconds cycle (high intensity)
90 seconds recovery
Repeat 3 times
2 minute cool-down and stretch out

Day 3

Run
3 minute warm-up
2 minute run (high intensity)
3 minute recovery
Repeat 3 times
5 minute cool-down and stretch out

Day 5

Circuits
3 minute warm-up
40 seconds squats
60 seconds recovery
40 seconds plank
60 seconds recovery
40 seconds lunges
60 seconds recover
30 seconds stairs
2 minute cool-down and stretch out

Diary Tracker

Use a diary to plan your programme and keep track of your progress, and to help you keep to your plan.

Activity and duration

Use the plans on pages 102–111 to begin your programme and as a guide. Then, adapt them. Adapt the duration of the exercises and play around with the recovery periods (but don't take them out), and add to the reps. Don't miss the important warm up or cool down periods. Keep each session short but intense.

Heart rate

You can regularly check your heart rate to see roughly at what level you are working (see page 22). Try not to let this interfere with the natural flow of your exercise. It's not going to be helpful to keep stopping after every two minutes to take your pulse. A heart monitor will give you an indication, but listen to your body. You will know when you are working hard, and when you need to ease up a little or push further.

Physical reaction

Noting down your physical reaction to your workout helps you think about how your body is responding to the challenge. You may need to change things slightly if it is too hard or add in more challenges if you need more of a challenge.

Feelings

Noting down how you feel will help you work out what you might need to change for the next week, or to plan differently so that it is more effective and enjoyable. The key to this exercise plan is to keep it working for you.

Appetite

It's useful to see if your appetite remains the same or whether it changes. Note down any changes in your diet.

Other changes

Other ways to measure your progress include your weight, waist measurement and how your clothes fit.

Targets

Plan ahead for the following week, giving yourself some targets to aim for. This might be trying your high intensity swim doing breaststroke instead of your favoured stroke, or cycling in a higher gear for part of your workout. Try to be realistic in your goals so that your fitness progress is measured and successful.

Be prepared to adapt to the other demands in your life – after all, this exercise is meant to work for you.

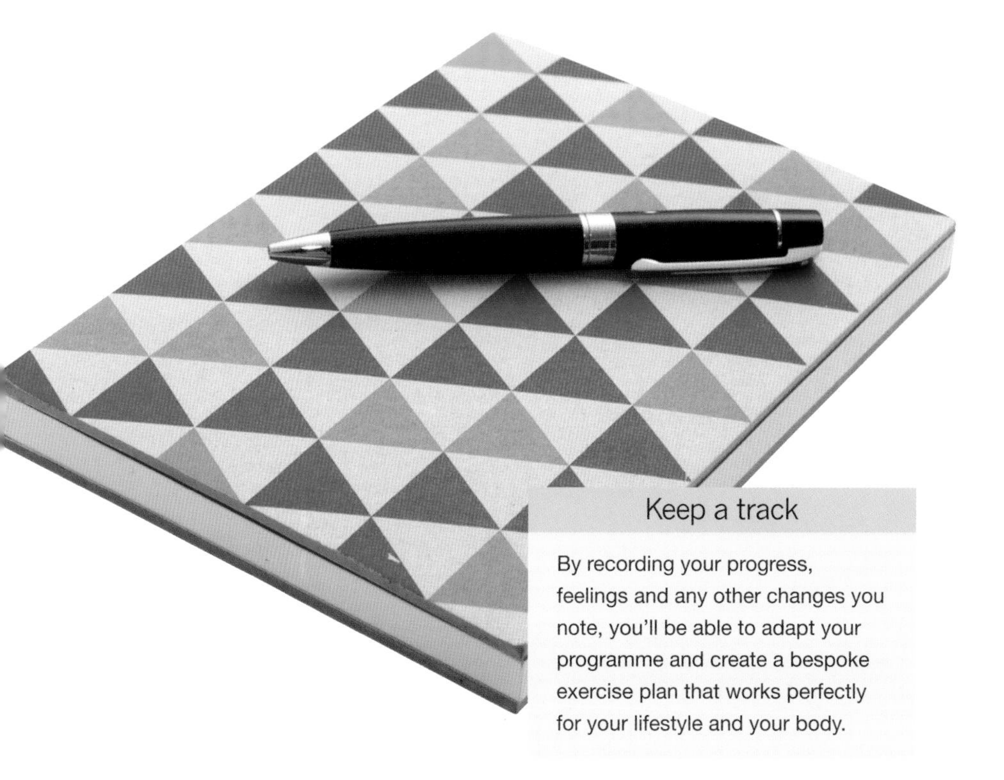

Keep a track

By recording your progress, feelings and any other changes you note, you'll be able to adapt your programme and create a bespoke exercise plan that works perfectly for your lifestyle and your body.

Week 1

	Day 1 Plan	Day 1 Actual	Day 2 Plan	Day 2 Actual	Day 3 Plan	Day 3 Actual
Warm-up						
Activity (and duration)						
Recovery						
Repetitions						
Cool-down						

	Notes	Notes	Notes
Heart rate level as %			
Other changes			
Physical reaction			
Feelings			
Appetite			
Targets			

Week 2

	Day 1 Plan	Day 1 Actual	Day 2 Plan	Day 2 Actual	Day 3 Plan	Day 3 Actual
Warm-up						
Activity (and duration)						
Recovery						
Repetitions						
Cool-down						

	Notes	Notes	Notes
Heart rate level as %			
Other changes			
Physical reaction			
Feelings			
Appetite			
Targets			

Week 3

	Day 1 Plan	Day 1 Actual	Day 2 Plan	Day 2 Actual	Day 3 Plan	Day 3 Actual
Warm-up						
Activity (and duration)						
Recovery						
Repetitions						
Cool-down						

	Notes	Notes	Notes
Heart rate level as %			
Other changes			
Physical reaction			
Feelings			
Appetite			
Targets			

Week 4

	Day 1 Plan	Day 1 Actual	Day 2 Plan	Day 2 Actual	Day 3 Plan	Day 3 Actual
Warm-up						
Activity (and duration)						
Recovery						
Repetitions						
Cool-down						

	Notes	Notes	Notes
Heart rate level as %			
Other changes			
Physical reaction			
Feelings			
Appetite			
Targets			

Week 5

	Day 1 Plan	Day 1 Actual	Day 2 Plan	Day 2 Actual	Day 3 Plan	Day 3 Actual
Warm-up						
Activity (and duration)						
Recovery						
Repetitions						
Cool-down						

	Notes	Notes	Notes
Heart rate level as %			
Other changes			
Physical reaction			
Feelings			
Appetite			
Targets			

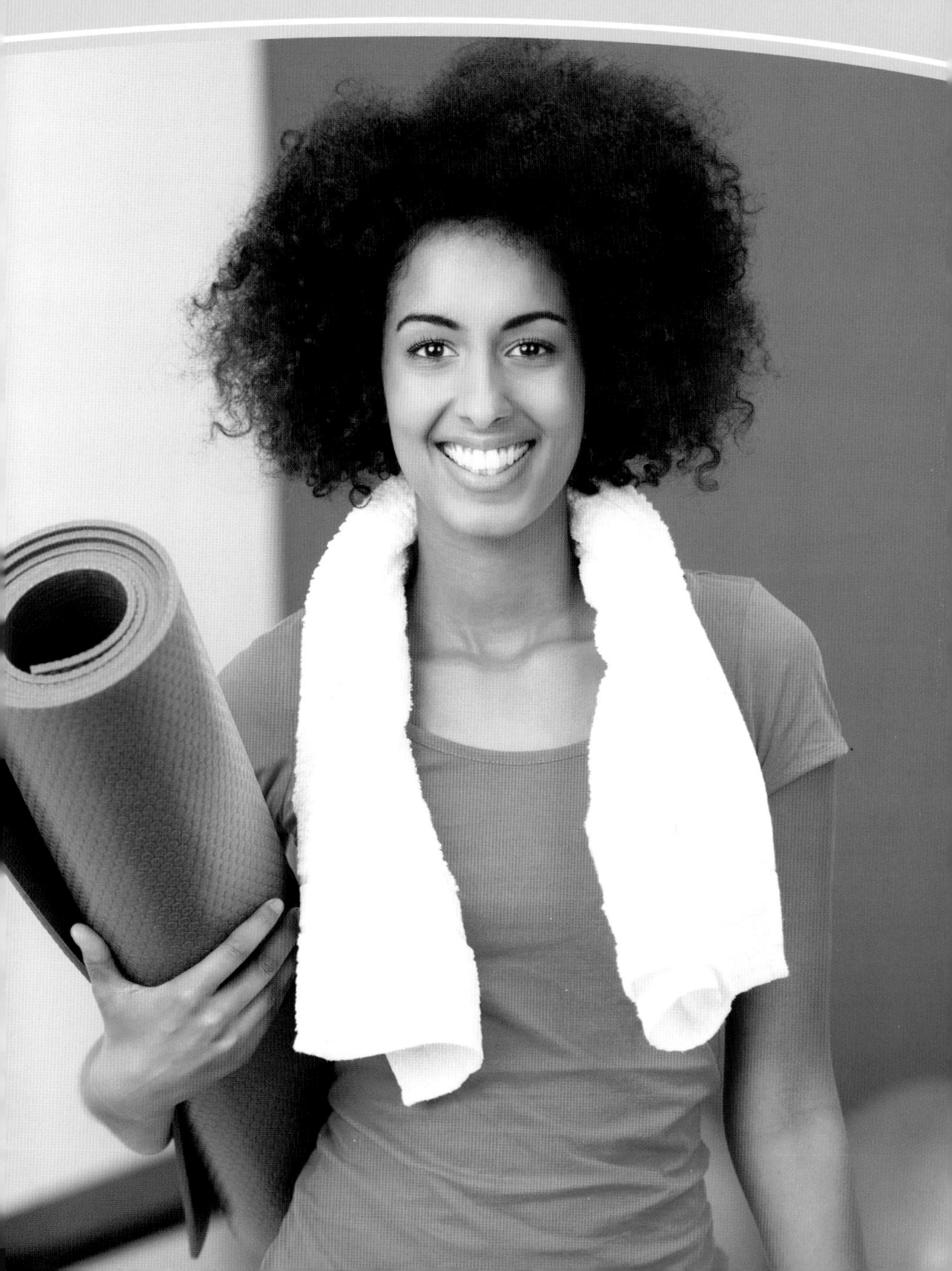

Major Muscles

Before embarking on any exercise plan, it is a good idea to understand where your muscles are so that you can work them effectively.

Arms

Biceps brachi – front of the upper arm
Brachialis – forearm
Brachioradialis – forearm
Deltoid – shoulders
Triceps brachi – back of the upper arm

Back

Latissimus dorsi – lower and middle back
Quadratus lumborum – lower back
Rhomboids – between the shoulder blades
Trapezius – upper middle and lower back

Abdominals

Internal and external *obliques* – waist
Rectus abdominus – front of ribs and pelvis
Transversus abdominus – deep in abdominal region

Hips and buttocks

Gluteus maximus – buttocks
Gluteus medius – side of buttocks
Gluteus minimus – side of buttocks
Ilipsoas – front of pelvis
Pectineus – front of the pubis

Legs

Adductor magnus, brevis and *longus* – inner thigh
Gastrocnemius and *soleus* – calf
Gracilis – inner thigh
Hamstring – back of leg
Quadriceps – front of thigh
Tibialis anterior – shin

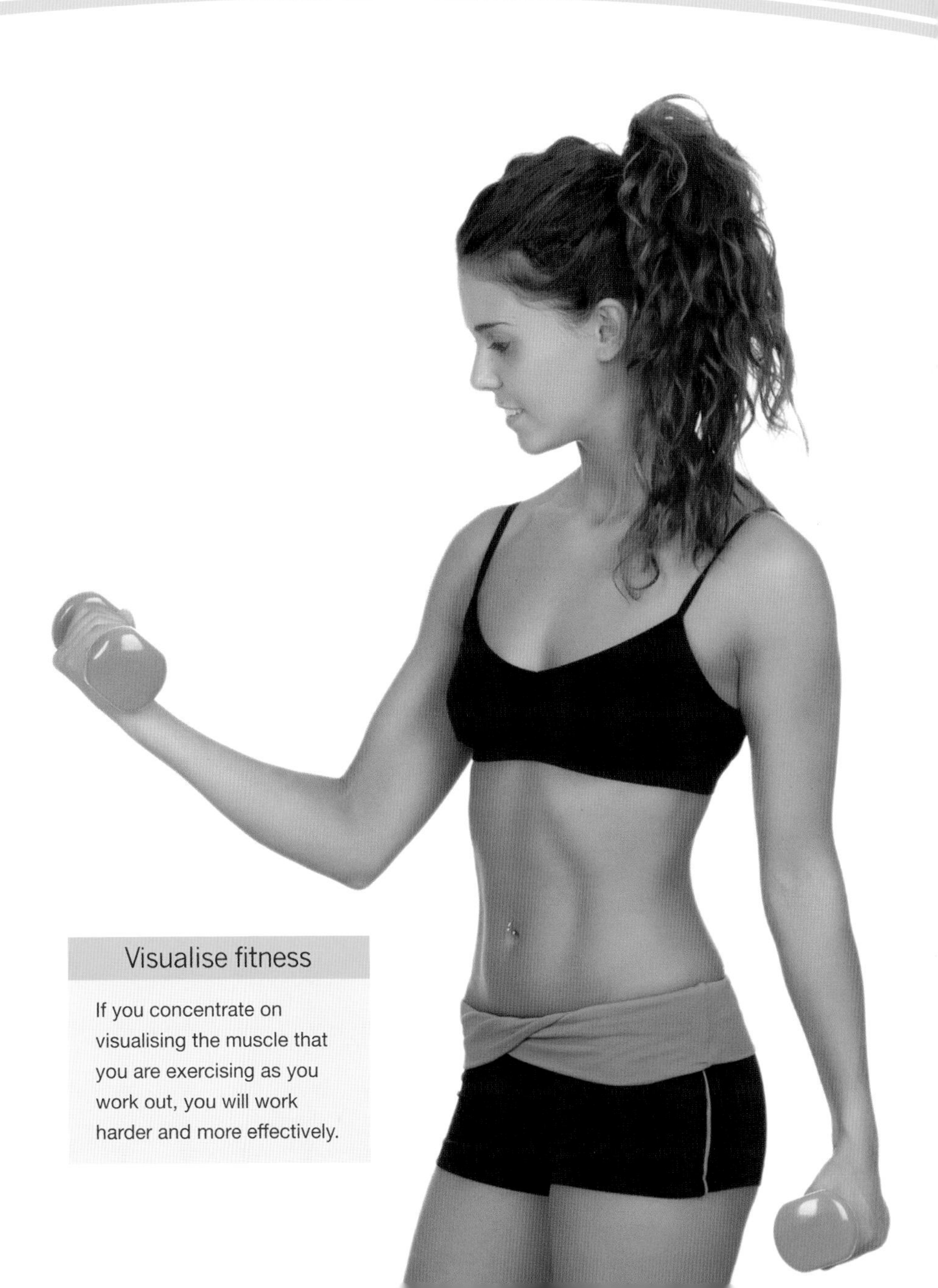

Visualise fitness

If you concentrate on visualising the muscle that you are exercising as you work out, you will work harder and more effectively.

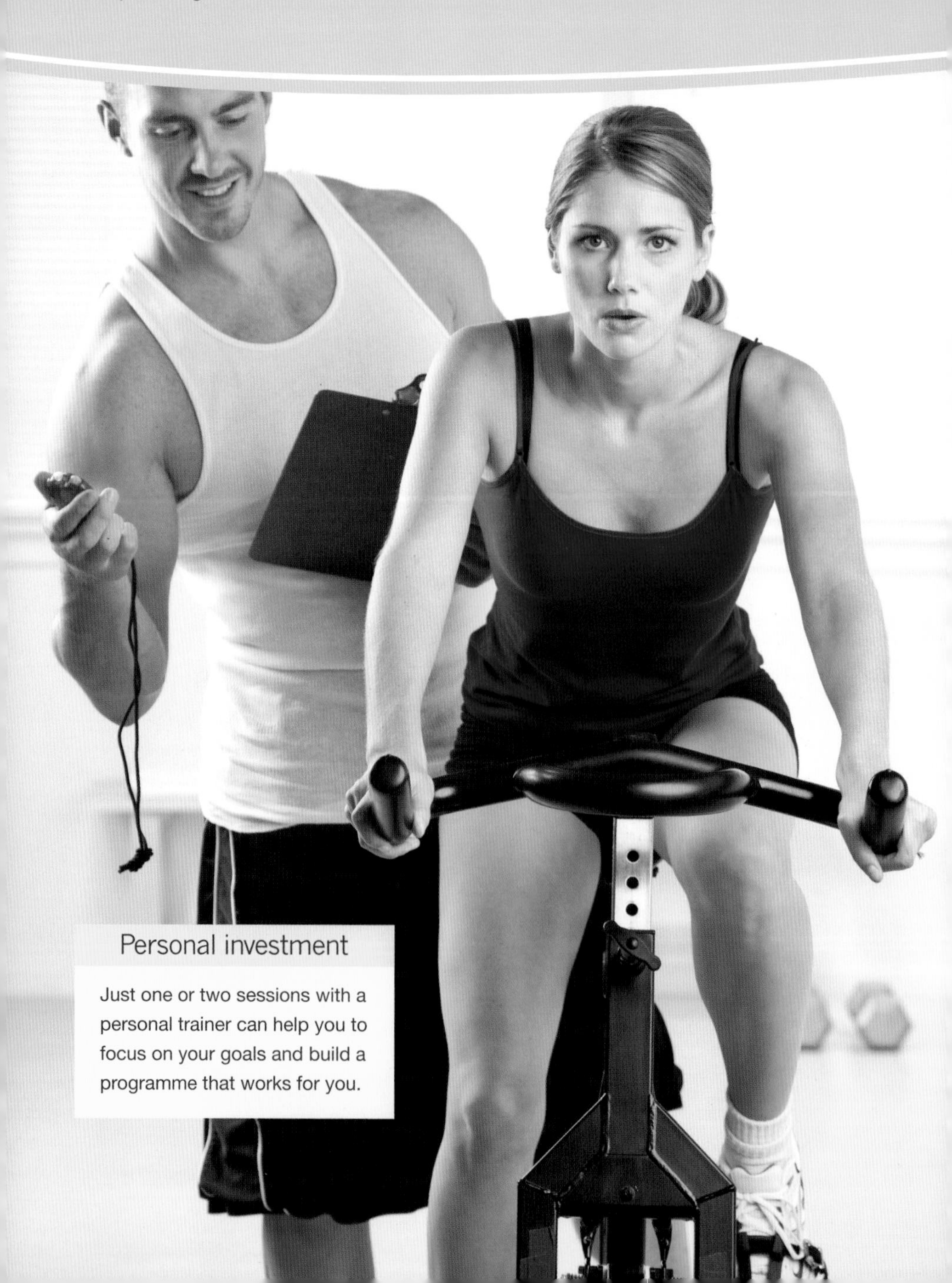

Personal investment

Just one or two sessions with a personal trainer can help you to focus on your goals and build a programme that works for you.

Keep It Fast

Frame fast fitness within an active life – don't just go for three minutes' high intensity as your week's exercise.

- Walk up the stairs rather than take a lift or the escalators
- Move around regularly when you are at work (especially if your job involves sitting at a desk)
- Put effort into any physical exercise – when you walk, walk with focus and energy. Keep your abdominals tight and your posture strong
- Join a running club or cycling group – make it social
- Play a team sport such as football, netball or badminton

Tech it

- Programme your exercise plan into your phone. That way it's always there to remind you
- Apps on phones or other devices are great at giving you instant exercise–calorie use calculations

Expertise

If you can, get the support of a trainer or coach. Share the cost with a group of friends. Treat yourself to a session with a nutritionist.

Keep progressing

Avoid the exercise plateau, where your body gets used to your regular exercise routine and you don't seem to lose any more weight or notice any other changes. Keep varying your high intensity work, making sure you are combining a range of activities. As you become more familiar with your workouts, check out different techniques. For instance, if you are going to try the butterfly stroke, look out for tips on techniques.

Fit for you

Adapt to your changes in life. Don't stress if your plan doesn't go exactly as you hoped. Say your bike gets a puncture: it's very annoying but rather than feel deflated or cross, do some intense bum and leg exercises at home instead – and then mend the puncture.

If you miss some days because of illness, then pick up when you are feeling better (and on your doctor's advice, if appropriate). Start off more gently than you otherwise would do. Build up to full strength and intensity.

Try to get someone to train with you from time to time, especially if you are running/cycling. You are more likely to stay on track and work hard.

On holiday or at work

Find a local park, or the beach is even better. Fast fitness is so easy to fit in because it takes minutes. It's not as if you are going to abandon family and friends for an hour every day!

You don't even need to pack weights – just buy some cans when you arrive.

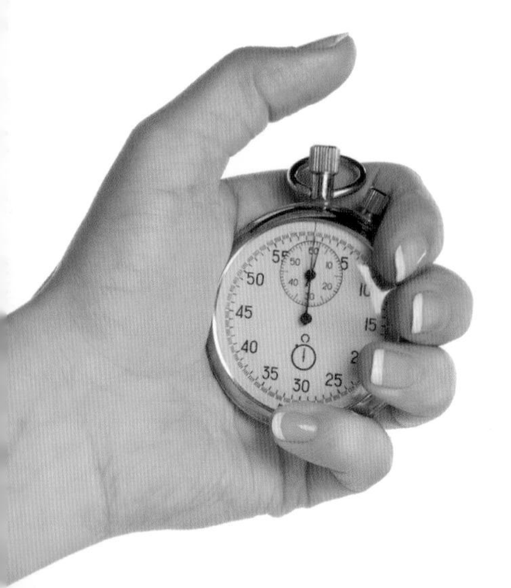

Use a timer

Counting seconds accurately is quite hard when your body is going at a certain pace, as the tendency is to count to the rhythm of your body. A stopwatch or timer will ensure that 20 seconds really is 20 seconds!

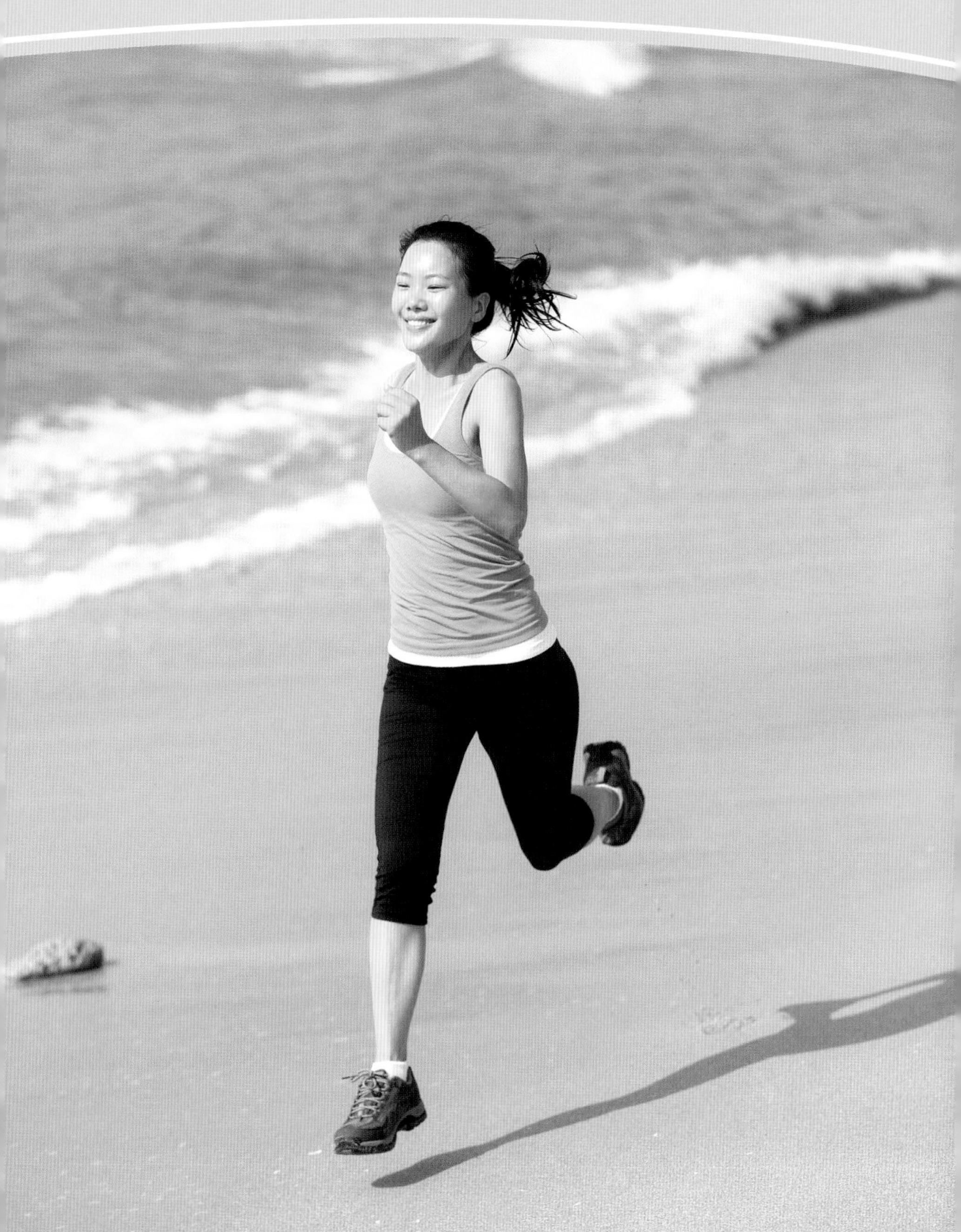

Motivate

One of the hardest aspects of exercise is keeping going. You start off with great intentions, but one setback or bad day, and the exercise plan is on the shelf.

These top tips will help you keep on top of your exercise plan, keep it going and keep you looking good and feeling great.

- Keep track of your progress – compare your fitness, feelings and look to the 'you' of a month previously
- Take pride in your efforts so far
- Enjoy how good you feel and look – enjoy your progress
- Reward yourself for your efforts

Secret tip

Chocolate milk… you may not have that at the top of your list of superfoods for exercising, but there is some research which shows that low fat chocolate milk is one of the best ways of replenishing a tired body with protein and carbs after a hard workout. It's either that or beet juice!

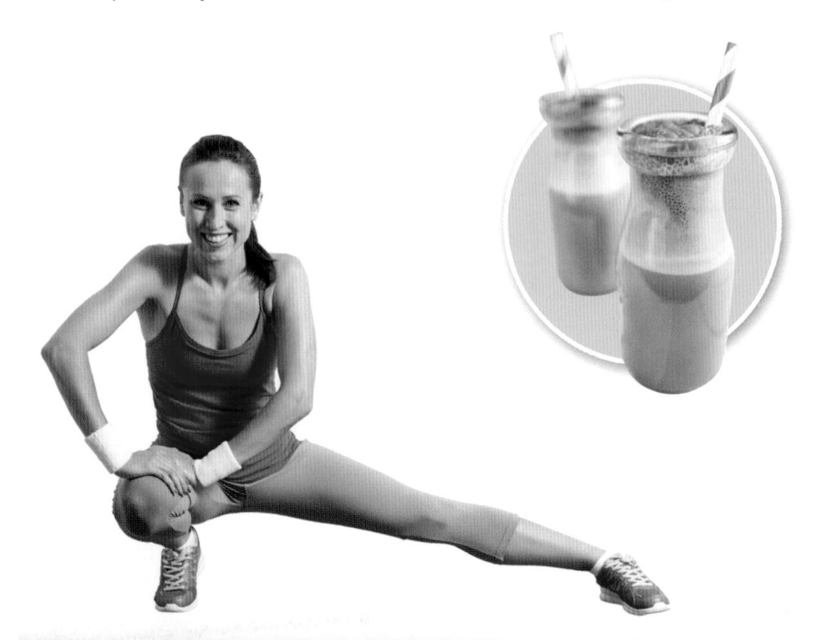

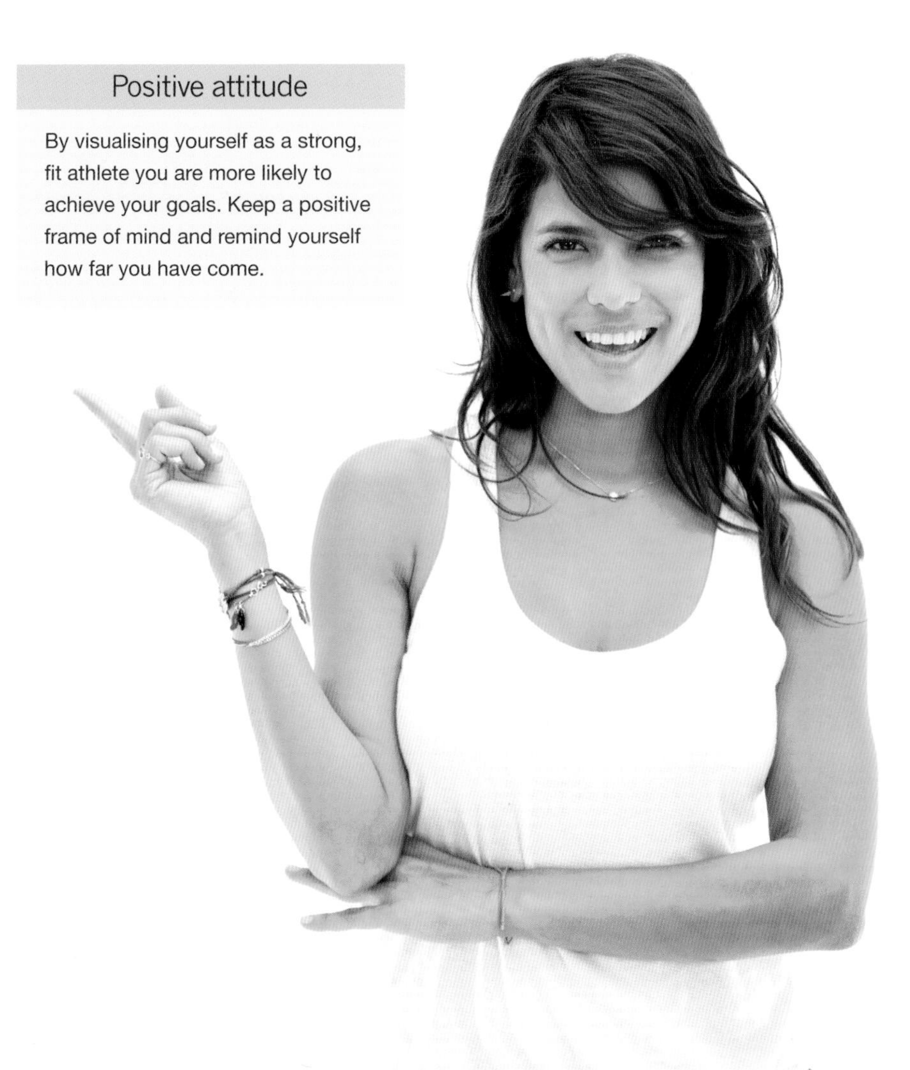

Positive attitude

By visualising yourself as a strong, fit athlete you are more likely to achieve your goals. Keep a positive frame of mind and remind yourself how far you have come.

Exercise consultant: Sandra Farnell.

All step-by-step exercise photography by Tudor Photography.

Cover: main Maridav/iStock; tl bennyartist/iStock; tc Picsfive/iStock; tr bogdandreava/iStock.

Flap: Thinkstock, Getty Images.

Picture Credits
4 Warren Goldswain/Shutterstock; 6 Andres Rodriguez/Dreamstime; 7 Hongmai2012/Dreamstime; 9 Ammentorp/Dreamstime; 10 Monkey Business Images/Dreamstime; 11t Pogonici/Dreamstime; 11b Vadymvdrobot/Dreamstime; 13 Martinmark/Dreamstime; 14 Andresr/Shutterstock; 17 Wavebreakmedia Ltd/Dreamstime; 19 Martinmark/Dreamstime; 20 Wavebreakmedia Ltd/Dreamstime; 23 Milenko Đilas/Dreamstime; 25 S_Photo/Shutterstock; 26 Martinmark/Dreamstime; 29 Warren Goldswain/Shutterstock; 31 Hongmai2012/Dreamstime; 44 Anna Kucherova/Dreamstime; 47 Nejron Photo/Shutterstock; 48 bikeriderlondon/Shutterstock; 51 Aleksandr Markin/Shutterstock; 52 Nejron/Dreamstime; 67 Pcheruvi/Dreamstime; 75 Sergiy Zavgorodny/Dreamstime; 86 Syda Productions/Shutterstock; 90 gresei/Shutterstock; 91 Dragonimages/Dreamstime; 92 Monkey Business Images/Dreamstime; 95 Stryjek/Dreamstime; 97 Hpphoto/Dreamstime; 98 Chesterf/Dreamstime; 100 wavebreakmedia/Shutterstock; 104 inxti/iStock; 105 Volodymyr Krasyuk/iStock; 106 Lai Leng Yiap/iStock; 111 Eliza317/iStock; 113 ChampCU/Shutterstock; 119 racorn/Shutterstock; 121 Jose Manuel Gelpi Diaz/Dreamstime; 122 Jonathan Ross/Dreamstime; 124 DenisNata/Shutterstock; 125 Uptall/Dreamstime; 126t Pinkcandy/Shutterstock; 126b ArtFamily/Shutterstock; 127 Andresr/Shutterstock; 128 Andres Rodriguez/Dreamstime.

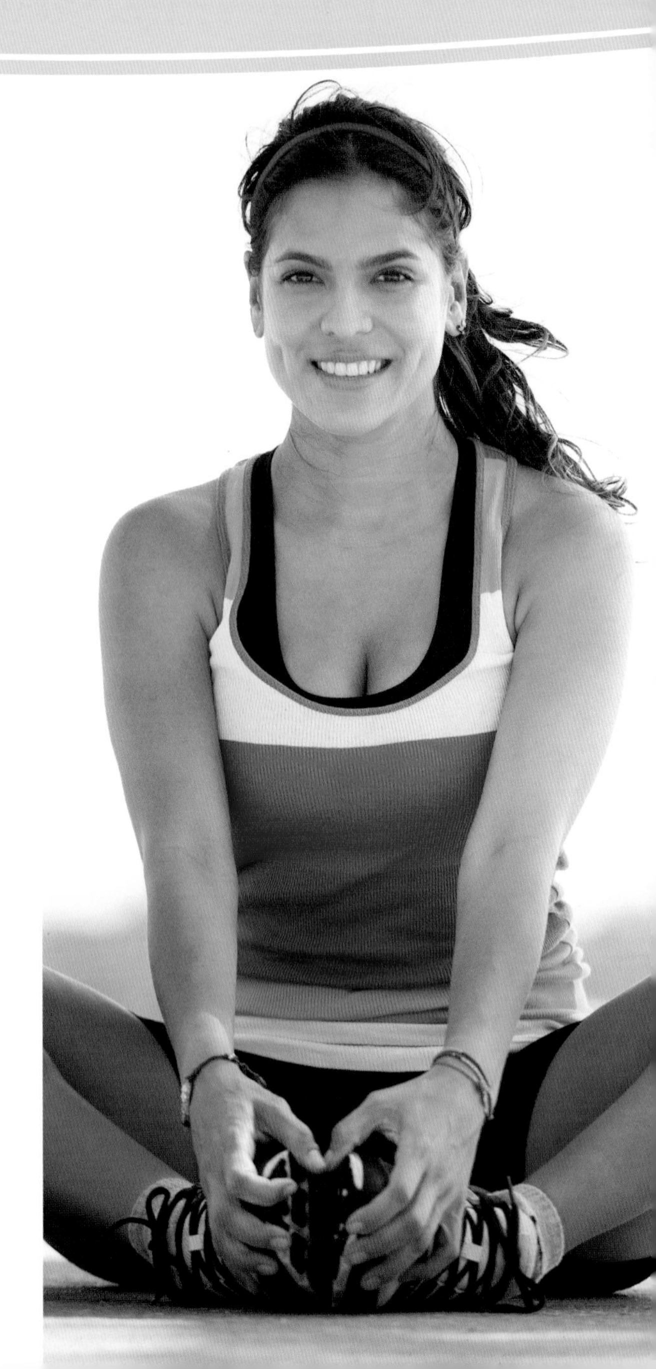